Community-Based Long-Term Care

Community-Based Long-Term Care

Innovative Models

Judith Ann Miller

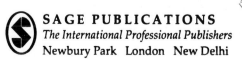

SAGE PUBLICATIONS
The International Professional Publishers
Newbury Park   London   New Delhi

For information address:

SAGE Publications, Inc.
2455 Teller Road
Newbury Park, California 91320

SAGE Publications Ltd.
6 Bonhill Street
London EC2A 4PU
United Kingdom

SAGE Publications India Pvt. Ltd.
M-32 Market
Greater Kailash I
New Delhi 110 048 India

Printed in the United States of America

Library of Congress Cataloging-in-Publication Data

Miller, Judith Ann.
    Community-based long-term care: innovative models / by Judith Ann
Miller.
        p.   cm.
    Materials from a study conducted for the Health Care Financing
Administration by a research team from the Center for Health
Services Research at the University of Colorado Health Sciences
Center.
    Includes bibliographical references.
    Includes indexes.
    ISBN 0-8039-3918-3 (c). — ISBN 0-8039-3919-1 (p.)
    1. Long-term care of the sick.   2. Community health services.
I. United States. Health Care Financing Administration.
II. University of Colorado Health Science Center. Center for Health
Services Research.   III. Title.
    [DNLM: 1. Community Health Services—organization &
administration—United States.   2. Long Term Care.   WT 30 M6485]
RA997.M523   1991
362.1'6—dc20
DNLM/DLC
for Library of Congress   90-9223
                                                                                                              CIP

FIRST PRINTING, 1991

Sage Production Editor: Michelle R. Starika

Contents

Preface

The primary purpose of this book is to present 12 successful models of community-based long-term health care. These programs are accessible for study and replication. It is hoped that students and teachers, administrators and directors, legislators and policymakers, clients, and families will find this information helpful as they work within the realm of planning and provision of long-term health care.

Research for this book began with a study conducted for the Health Care Financing Administration (HCFA) as part of its response to congressional mandates contained in the Medicare Catastrophic Coverage Act of 1988 (P.L. 100-360). The purpose of the study was to review past and current research and to provide recommendations on future research in two areas: (a) the quality of community-based and custodial long-term care services and (b) the relationship between long-term care (LTC) services and acute-care expenditures. The study was conducted by a research team at the Center for Health Services Research at the University of Colorado Health Sciences Center in Denver, Colorado.

Several comprehensive reports resulted from the project, including Schlenker, Miller, Berg, Bischof, and Butler (1989) and Miller, Berg, Bischoff, and Schlenker (1989), and have been passed on to the HCFA for further study. However, after the reports were written, there was a considerable amount of valuable information that would not be filed away. A number of successful community-based long-term health care programs, some of which are described in this book, were discovered to have met the challenges of providing quality care within a complex system of fragmented funding and uncoordinated services.

AUTHOR'S NOTE: The statements contained in this book are solely those of the authors and do not necessarily reflect the views or policies of the Health Care Financing Administration or the Center for Health Services Research, University of Colorado Health Sciences Center, Denver, Colorado.

These innovative programs have developed as a result of much planning, brainstorming, cooperation, caring, and tenacity. The leaders of such programs have each agreed to coauthor a chapter in this book regarding their respective programs in order to present some of their experiences and success tips.

Community-Based Long-Term Care: Innovative Models is organized into two sections, the first of which includes an introduction to programmatic issues facing the long-term care health system. A complete description of services, caregivers, payers, and licensure/certification regulations are presented. Section II then describes twelve models for community-based long-term health care, including its service delivery system.

SUMMARY OF SERVICES, PAYERS, AND REGULATIONS

An introduction to community-based long-term home health care will assist the reader in understanding the makeup and delivery of home care. A taxonomy and definition of all services are offered and are followed by a description of payers and the services encompassed by each payer. Regulation, certification, and accreditation of services also are listed. Each service, regulation, and payer has a long history too involved to fully describe in this brief overview. However, it is hoped that this introduction will serve as a base to illustrate how each model has drawn from the past to create a system of comprehensive care for the present and future.

INNOVATIVE MODELS FOR COMMUNITY-BASED HEALTH CARE

Twelve selected models for community-based long-term health care are described in Section II. Each model has innovatively coordinated several service segments and met the challenge of creating a successful service-delivery system. The history of development and philosophy of each program, as well as a full description of the service delivery system, is presented.

The chapters have been coauthored by the directors/developers of the models and represent their many years of experience. As the biographies indicate, the coauthors are well-educated professionals who share a common mission of "caring about long-term care." Another commonality is that each has taken what has been successful from traditional service systems and has drawn from an innovative vision to create a unique system of comprehensive care. I was fortunate to have visited several of the model facilities and programs and am honored to have worked with these cooperative, enthusiastic pioneers.

Judith A. Miller

Introduction

The availability of service is the greatest challenge to home care in the 1990s. Home care is rapidly becoming capacity constrained; personnel are becoming scarce and unit cost is increasing. Meeting the requisite of serving the right people at the right time with the right service will be very difficult unless some fundamental changes are initiated within the home-care delivery system (Foley, 1989).

During the 1980s, developing long-term care systems has been a crucial concern among policymakers, providers, consumers, and researchers. The home-care industry has expanded considerably, not only in terms of volume of funding, provider agencies, and clients, but also in the range of services available. These wheels of progress have been driven by two forces: the ever-expanding older segment of the population requiring these services, and a national effort to prevent early or unnecessary institutionalization of the elderly and disabled (LTC Management, 1989b).

The Graying of America. The population at risk for long-term care is expanding at a phenomenal rate. It is projected that by 2030, there will be 12 million frail, elderly Americans.

Policy to Reduce Institutionalization. If disability rates persist, it is projected that the number of elderly entering nursing homes will more than triple from 1.3 million in 1984 to 5.3 million in 2030. Alternative approaches to care delivery and financing could significantly alter the need for institutionalized care (Holahan & Sulvetta, 1989).

Innovation in funding and service delivery is necessary to meet these needs as the home-care industry continues to demand more effectual/proficient planning. In order to plan for effective, efficient service delivery, it is essential to understand the nature of care needs, the resources consumed in care delivery, and the characteristics of patients receiving care (Phillips, Applebaum, Atchley, & McGinnis, 1989).

1

The Nature of Care. Regarding understanding the nature of care needs, Montgomery (1989) distinguished three dimensions of health functioning: functional limitations (i.e., reduction in patient's capacity to perform self-care); cognitive status, including memory and judgment impairments; and global health status, an overall evaluation of the frail elder's physical health. Each dimension or combination of functioning levels could directly affect the process and cost of care.

Hughes (1989) also notes that long-term-care clients have multiple, chronic conditions and require care over an extended period of time in varied environments. Therefore, Hughes suggests that comprehensive, multidimensional methods determine a "degree of risk" index that would consider the technical complexity of needs, service setting, and degree of frailty of the client to prescribe the level of care required.

The commonality of these reports is the implication of the need for the development of patient-classification systems to describe and measure clinical care, counseling, and coordination of all care services. Phillips and Miller (1987) suggest that these community-care, case-mix considerations revolve around several significant issues: nonreimbursed care; a more comprehensive case management component; family caretakers; and resource requirements and distribution. These interrelated issues are presented below.

NONREIMBURSED CARE

In an attempt to quantify amount and types of nonbilled home care, Phillips, Scattergood, Fisher, and Baglioni (1988) found that reimbursed care represents a small portion of the care that is required and delivered. With a sample of 350 Virginia public, home-health patient episodes, the researchers reviewed billing records to determine the number of billed home visits per episode. Home-health records were then matched, and all visits and care-related activities (i.e., phone calls, conferences, laboratory trips) were recorded. The results indicated an increase of total home visits, with an average of 1.5 unbilled home visits per episode. In addition there were 10 unbilled care-related activities per patient.

These changing trends of less care per case are occurring at a time when patients needing home care have more complex and diverse needs than ever before. A secondary trend is that of private and proprietary agencies referring patients with inadequate potential for reimbursement to the public service sector, thereby impressing strain on an already overburdened and underfunded system.

Home Health Resource Consumption. Traditionally, studies of home-health consumption have tracked utilization via billing records. It is believed that much more care is actually delivered than is billed or reimbursed and that relying solely on billing records will severely underestimate utilization and will further restrict anticipated prospective payment in home health care.

Patient Outcomes. Coordination of agencies and services, as well as home health aide visits following skilled nursing termination, can be critically essential to long-term homecare patients. Over the years, home health nurses have created practice patterns based on professional judgment about patient and family needs.

Careful consideration should be given to the consequences of nonreimbursed care on patient outcome and quality of care.

Shifting Mix of Patients. A pilot study of public home health found an increase in nonreimbursable care and a resource consumption shift from an acute/chronic mix of patients to almost exclusively chronic/long-term patients (Phillips & Miller, 1987). A second shift due to changes in home health care reimbursement has been the growth in private-sector agencies. This has resulted in a split in the kinds of persons served by public and private agencies. For example, public agencies tend to provide more frequent visits for longer periods of time (Medicare and indigent), while private agencies have much greater flexibility in the types of clients (paying) they wish to accept and types of services (reimbursable) they wish to provide.

If these concurrent trends (prioritization of home care and patterns of chronic long-term care) continue, three questions must be considered. First, because current reimbursement primarily reflects acute-care services, how will complex, chronic care be delivered and reimbursed? Second, what will happen to chronically ill patients with nonreimbursable needs? Third, will the "quicker and sicker" hospital discharges conflict with the needs and resources for the growing population of chronically ill?

COMPREHENSIVE CASE MANAGEMENT

Anticipatory surveillance best describes the future role of case managers. The success of future case management is dependent upon the development of standards for service and long-term care case management, both of which are currently loosely defined and not widely regulated. Case management goals must include both cost-containment and quality-assurance mechanisms. They must maximize the functional independence and quality of life for disabled individuals. There must be equity and efficiency in the allocation of long-term care resources (Lyons, 1989a).

Cost Containment. A cost-of-care measure is a necessary case-management tool designed for screening patient needs. It helps the case manager to determine a care plan that considers consequences to care providers (especially family caregivers) in terms of costs.

Quality Assurance. In addition to economic costs, it is necessary to measure the value of care provision, personal restrictions, social disruptions, the care recipient as provocateur, and psychosomatic consequences.

FAMILY CARE SYSTEM

Care must be taken in placing a patient in the informal or family care system. Many families can serve as an effective care system for their elders, but other family systems represent an inappropriate choice for caregiving. For example, a patient's spouse may be functionally limited or impaired to some degree, or a son/daughter may be an alcoholic, be unemployed, or not have a suitable living arrangement for caregiving.

Case managers must consider the family or informal caregiver's economic, physical, psychological, and social resources. Therefore, a dual assessment is needed: one to consider the patient, and another to determine the feasibility of the patient's family in the caregiver role.

The Family Resource Assessment. The family assessment process places the case manager in a double bind as a care plan is drawn. First, as the coordinator of resources necessary to meet the patient needs, the family has the potential to fulfill the majority of needs and account for the majority of the care cost. Second, the case manager fulfills the patient-protection role in assessing the family caregiver's ability to adequately perform the caregiving services, or, conversely, considering the potential danger of abuse and neglect if a patient were inappropriately placed in a dysfunctional family setting. The case manager thus must employ the essential assessments to make the proper decision in the development of a collaborative and cooperative relationship between the formal and informal support systems.

All models described herein view case management as the core of their program, essentially maintaining the family as the primary support system. Its purpose is to eliminate fragmentation and duplication of patient services; to assure continuity of services; to closely monitor all aspects of patient care; to observe changes in condition or unmet needs; to afford the patient and family the security of after-hours and weekend services; to facilitate a close and positive relationship with the patient; and to order the most appropriate and cost-effective patient care. These elements maintain and enhance the family support system.

RESOURCE REQUIREMENTS AND DISTRIBUTION

There is a critical need for better-designed programs to meet the differential levels of home care. They must be targeted at various types of patients and the length of service in relation to the effectiveness and cost of home care. This process will include the development of services better and less expensive than institutionalization for each type of chronically ill patient, and the targeting of these services to ensure that the needs of patients and the services delivered are appropriately equated (Hedrick & Inui, 1986).

INNOVATIVE, COMPREHENSIVE CASE-MANAGED SERVICE MODELS

The models presented in this book are examples of programs strategically designed to meet the above-mentioned goals and needs. They were specifically selected because they appear to be better and less expensive than institutionalization and provide the most appropriate type of care for each client.

Model Similarities

Although each program is distinctively unique, they all share common threads. These commonalities are listed and described below within the format of presentation: program description, philosophy, history of development, service delivery, financial component, evaluation, and replication.

Program Descriptions. All models grew from a small seed in some caring person's mind and were nurtured by a concerned community. Many programs had their beginnings at a kitchen table over a cup of coffee. Because there was a growing need, a service system was developed and implemented to meet that need. Community-based care is two-sided; while care is provided to the elderly, the community works diligently to assure continuity of care. These models are at various stages of growth but are deemed successful and replicable.

Philosophy. The value of home and the family is the underlying stimulus of each program. Quality of life and cost containment are dual considerations in providing service that will allow clients the choice to remain in their own home or home-like environment for as long as possible. Each program is designed to enhance the ability of a family to meet the needs of its elderly.

History of Development. Each program has grown slowly over the past decade. One step at a time has been the common growth pattern, and each step has involved considerable and careful planning by a concerned community, legislators, health care providers, and clients. Parallel social, economic, and political aspects have been orchestrated in an innovative manner. The success of these programs has been contingent upon cooperation and committed work toward a shared vision. The history of each program is meant to be a composite lesson for those interested in duplicating or developing programs.

Service Delivery. A wide array of services and a multidisciplinary care system have been designed and developed within each program. Family caregivers are a vital part of all models, and respite care is a service provided to relieve the family burden of care. Each model also has a volunteer element essential to service delivery and cost containment.

Financial Component. Fragmented funding has been coordinated to correlate with a comprehensive service system. Each program relies heavily on the family as a care unit and provides respite care to support the family. Volunteers also contribute to the financial component, and communities and legislators are committed to success. Although funding is limited, each program speaks to cost-effective care delivery.

Evaluation. Close scrutiny has been a constant in each phase of development, and continued evaluation is a vital element of present and future service planning. Several models have gained national recognition and distinguished awards.

Replication. Expansion and replication efforts for each project are explained and presented for study and consideration by other agencies, communities, or states wishing to duplicate programs in the quest for finding workable community-based services for the elderly and disabled.

IN-HOME PROGRAMS

Respite Care Center (Evanston, Illinois)

Most long-term care for the elderly is provided by family members at great personal and financial sacrifice. Because of the pivotal importance of families in helping to maintain disabled elderly persons at home, the interest in family caregivers for dependent elders is a primary concern. Respite care differs from other long-term care programs in that it serves dual clients: the older person in need of care, and the caregiver who needs breakaway time from the burden of care. Many of the models described in this book include respite care in their array of services, but one program in particular is receiving worldwide attention: the Respite Care Center of Evanston, Illinois. It serves as a model of respite care that stands alone or can be incorporated into a more comprehensive program that offers a variety of services.

The Respite Care Center of Evanston, Illinois, is presented as a model utilizing volunteers to deliver support services focused on the caregiver. This center provides temporary relief from the responsibility of caring for a physically and/or cognitively dependent individual. The program's goal is to sustain the caregiving relationship, thereby enabling the elderly individual to remain in the home or community setting. The project encompasses a comprehensive array of services, including in-home and institutional-based respite care, information and referral, case management, client advocacy, and community and professional education activities. Central to the nurse-managed respite care project is the referral of family caregivers to existing community resources, and case management services to families enrolled in the respite program. Community-based respite services in the home are provided by both trained volunteers and paid home respite workers.

Five Hospital Homebound Elderly Program
(Chicago, Illinois)

Despite the common view that most elderly live in nursing homes, only about 5% of the elderly do so at any given time. The vast majority live quietly in their own homes and apartments, often forgotten and abandoned. Five North Side Chicago hospitals (Columbus-Cabrini Medical Center, Grant Hospital of Chicago, Saint Joseph Hospital, and Health Care Center) are to be commended for cooperating and coordinating a home-care program to provide home health services as an alternative to hospitalization or nursing home placement for homebound, chronically ill elderly neighbors.

The Five Hospital Program has been selected as a model for consideration by other large cities. Rather than have each hospital form its own separate program, the consolidation of staff, financial resources, administration, and all other program components has been a key to successful service. Five Hospital provides a continuity of care to the homebound by utilizing a multidisciplinary team of health care professionals and volunteers in accordance with an individual plan of care for each patient. Within the program's capacity, it provides charity care to individuals regardless of their ability to pay.

There are short-term and long-term components to this mission. Short-term care allows patients to recover at home after a prior hospitalization. Long-term care enables elderly clients to live out their lives in dignity at home. By taking advantage of community support systems, patients avoid chronic neglect, frequent hospitalization, and unnecessary premature institutionalization.

The Block Nurse Program (St. Paul, Minnesota)

The cornerstone of the Block Nurse Program is the enhancement of the ability of a family to meet the needs of its members and is based on the premise that keeping people at home and out of institutions enhances their quality of life, enriches neighborhoods, and reduces costs.

The award-winning model has been selected because it combines innovation and resourcefulness. The Block Nurse Program, a joint venture between the local government entity and the Public Health Nursing Service, is an innovative departure from the conventional service delivery system. This decentralized model is a promising example of how community initiative can redesign service delivery for the frail elderly to provide more effective care at less cost. Block Nurse has a neighborhood focus, drawing upon professional and volunteer residents living in the neighborhood to provide home health and long-term care for elderly and disabled neighbors.

After seven years of providing services to elderly clients, the Block Nurse Program has found that cost-effective services can be delivered based upon the elderly's needs rather than eligibility for reimbursement. What is required is alternative funding; professional and volunteer community members; and an informal network of family, friends, neighbors, churches, civic groups, and service clubs, such as Boy Scouts and Rotary clubs.

Rural Elderly Enhancement Program
(Montgomery, Alabama)

Another model of community involvement can be found in Alabama and is targeted at two of the poorest counties of the nation. The Rural Elderly Enhancement program is a nurse-managed project, the purpose of which is to implement a community-involved organization and infrastructure development (housing, water, transportation) to improve the health and quality of life of rural, poor elderly who live in isolated areas and lack transportation. The program has created community coalitions to respond to the elderly's needs by linking services, training, respite care, and education. The coalitions work as a cooperative effort with community agencies and indigenous residents to serve as advocates for the elderly and their caregivers.

Outcomes of the project include the enhancement of independent living for the elderly; collaboration among community agencies; personal empowerment of the elderly residents and county residents; training and job placement for low-income residents; and infrastructure improvement (water, housing, and transportation).

Wyoming Community-Based In-Home Services Program
(Cheyenne, Wyoming)

A Social Model for Community-Based In-Home Services for the Profoundly Rural Elderly is a rural-social model that relies on paraprofessional case managers who operate under the direction of program directors based in multipurpose senior centers. At a time when both human and financial resources for home health care are limited, Wyoming has created a program to provide quality care to a widely dispersed elderly population.

The program began in 1985 with four pilot projects. At the time this book went to press, the program has expanded to 23 county-based programs, with major goals directed at enabling the elderly, especially the frail elderly, to remain at home and minimize their vulnerability to premature institutionalization. The key component in Wyoming's rural-social model is the cooperative relationship among paraprofessional case managers, primary care providers, and members of other private and voluntary sectors within a community in the delivery and monitoring of services. The program's accountability depends on total client involvement in making choices and evaluating outcomes and in paying their fair share of services.

PASSPORT (State of Ohio)

PASSPORT is a model in which case managers combine client pre-assessment and care planning to deliver appropriate care. These two components are the Pre-Admission Screening System (PASS) and Providing Options and Resources Today (PORT). The program grew from the national Channeling Demonstration sponsored by HCFA in the early 1980s to a statewide program designed to slow the growth of Ohio's long-term care spending, to dramatically expand the availability of community-based long-term care, and to provide persons with long-term care needs with options whenever possible. Case management is clearly a key component to the PASSPORT intervention. The case manager's responsibility is to make sense out of a complex, fragmented service system, ensuring adequate linkage of client needs and services. It is the responsibility of the case manager to continually monitor the client's condition and the services provided.

Nursing Home Without Walls (State of New York)

As its name denotes, the Nursing Home Without Walls (NHWW) provides nursing-home-level care to patients in their homes rather than requiring them to be institutionalized. The program was developed in 1977 by New York State Senator Tarky Lombardi, Jr., as an alternative to long-term institutionalization. New York has developed a statewide program that serves an integral role in the state's long-term care system, which provides and coordinates the delivery of comprehensive services to the chronically ill and disabled so they may be cared for at home. The program's conception, growth, and development is described in chapter 10. NHWW has clearly demonstrated that it meets patients' needs in a less costly and more desirable setting—that is to say, the patient's own home. Serving as a pioneer in the nation's community-based care initiative, NHWW promises to continue to be a major force in meeting the increasing challenges of long term care and in shaping and directing the future of such care.

The Connecticut Hospice, Inc.
(Branford, Connecticut)

The first hospice in the United States, the Connecticut Hospice, Inc., was selected as a model for this book and is patterned after the first modern hospice founded in London in 1967. The purpose of hospice is to encourage the quality and comfort of existence for the patient and family, to enhance life for as long as it lasts. Because hospice generally is provided for only a few months, it is not necessarily a long-term service. However, in many cases it is a service coordinated with other long-term programs and often is the last service in a client's life.

Connecticut Hospice offers in-home service, hospital service, and live-in programs. This hospice's volunteerism, an integral part of the program, has gained national acclaim. On August 16, 1990, President George Bush designated the volunteers of The Connecticut Hospice as the 223rd Point of Light in his quest for 1,000 Points of Light marking personal service on behalf of others.

ASSISTED LIVING PROGRAMS

Generations Assisted Living Homes
(Duluth, Minnesota)

The Generations Model of long-term care specializes in offering assisted living in normal homes for persons with Alzheimer's disease and related conditions. These homes are licensed, adult, foster care and are structured to access funding for low-income (Medicaid-eligible) individuals. The program is presented herein as a generic model with wide applicability for both older and younger persons who are "at risk" of institutionalization. The model is service integrated, combining the services of adult foster care and personal care, and is financially sound and self-sufficient based on program earnings.

Concepts in Community Living (Portland, Oregon)

A social model of care, Concepts in Community Living successfully supports very frail individuals in residential settings. A 24-hour staff is available to provide care and service on an as-needed basis. This built-in service allows more impaired, frail people to continue living in a homelike environment. The overall goal is not to have a standard service package, but to maintain the capability to deliver basic services to all residents, on an individual basis, at all times. A monthly evaluation of service needs, with adjustments in the level and cost of service, allows a successful implementation of the "aging in place" concept for a frail population. This model of assisted living is a successful merger of housing and long-term care services.

INTEGRATED PROGRAMS

On Lok Senior Health Services
(San Francisco, California)

The On Lok Senior Health Services is a consolidated model of long-term care that has developed an innovative service and financial system for caring for the impaired elderly. The capitated model began as a demonstration program and has evolved to replication demonstration programs throughout the United States. No other community-based program in the United States offers all supportive and medical (both acute and chronic) services through the same program, reimbursed by both Medicare and Medicaid capitation payments.

Total Longterm Care (Denver, Colorado)

Total Longterm Care (TLC) provides health care services within an adult day health center for those elderly who are at risk of nursing home placement. The mission of the program is to promote the ability of the frail elderly to live in the community with dignity and independence. As an alternative to long-term nursing home placement, TLC maintains participants in their own homes for as long as possible and provides support for family caregivers. The program is a replication of On Lok, a PACE (Program of All-Inclusive Care for the Elderly) demonstration project. PACE is coordinating the replication initiative for Total Long-term Care and other such programs across the nation. Each replication project is designed to be as similar as possible to On Lok, but unique characteristics of the replication site determine the variances that must be considered.

As TLC is a demonstration project, its success is yet to be determined. However, the purpose of the demonstration is to determine whether the model (On Lok replication) can succeed outside San Francisco. Populations, state environments, geography of the city, and cultural and generational attitudes will influence the success of the site. The proof will unfold as the Denver site continues to implement the model in its own unique way.

EXPANSION OR REPLICATION

All models presented are considered replicable; in fact, many of them are currently in replication. Most chapters in this book have been coauthored by the program's director in order to present the models as accurately and completely as possible and to give the reader reference to a person who can serve as a consultant in replication planning.

SECTION I

Community-Based Long-Term Care

1

Caregivers and
Array of Services

Community-based long-term health care is defined as that component of comprehensive health care in which services are provided to individuals and families in the home for the purpose of promoting or restoring health or minimizing the effects of illness and disability. Services appropriate for the needs of the individual client and family are planned and coordinated by an agency using employed staff or contractual agreements. Community-based long-term care differs from nursing-home care in that services are provided to persons living at home or in home-like environments rather than to residents of institutions.

Scope and Content of Services. A striking characteristic of the community-based service area is the imprecision surrounding its scope and content. Many different terms are used to denote the general cluster of services involved. Despite the variety of definitions, community-based care usually connotes services provided to frail elderly and to disabled persons of all ages. The main objectives of the services are to assist clients with basic living tasks or to provide relief to their caregivers.

Community-based services thus cover a wide array of services, ranging from skilled-level medically related ones to social support services typically provided by paraprofessionals and informal caregivers. The skilled-level medically related services are funded primarily by Medicare and to some extent by Medicaid. Medicaid also covers certain of the support services, as do other public and private sources.

In general, the formal (i.e., paid) community-based services complement or support services provided by family members and informal caregivers. About 75% of the disabled elderly who live outside an institution rely solely on informal care (U.S. Senate, 1988b). Paid caregiving is a last resort for most dependent elderly. According to the 1982 Long-Term Care Survey, only 5% of community-based long-term care recipients receive all of their care from paid sources, and only 25% of paid long-term care in the community is financed through government sources.

Primary Caregivers. The majority of primary caregivers are either wives or adult daughters. According to numerous studies, about 86% of informal caregivers help with shopping and transportation, 81% with household tasks, and 76% with one or more personal hygiene activities. About half of caregivers help with transportation, administer medications, or handle financial matters. On the average, caregivers spend approximately 4 hours per day on such tasks. In addition, informal caregivers serve as links to formal, paid services for the disabled elderly.

A national survey of caregivers conducted by the American Association of Retired Persons, or AARP (1988) also reported that most (85%) long-term care is provided by family members, with at least 5 million Americans providing care to a parent or spouse at any given time. The survey profiled these caregivers as mostly minority women who must balance the demands of caregiving with paid employment. One in 10 provide round-the-clock care; at the least, one third have been providing care for more than 6 years. Family caregivers provide intensive physical, financial, and emotional support, with 50% spending at least 12 hours per day on caregiving. The survey revealed that formal services support family care rather than supplant it: Families use home-care aides and day care to extend home care and defray nursing home placement (AARP, 1988).

Taxonomy of Services. The task of classifying community-based long-term care is "a reflection of the piecework and patchwork of long-term care" (Kane & Kane, 1987, p.164). For purposes of explaining these models, a taxonomy of services and key caregivers are listed in Table 1.1.

Five main categories of services are listed:

1. assessment, information, and referral services that include services that help persons find and coordinate home care;
2. health and support services that include medically related home care and personal and custodial in-home care;
3. community-based out-of-home services provided outside the home;

Table 1.1 Taxonomy of Community-Based Long-Term Health Care
Service Domain

Assessment/Information/Referral Related Services
Case Management
Geriatric Assessment Services
Hospital Discharge Planning
Information and Referral

Health and Support Services

Medically-Related	*Personal and Custodial In-Home*
Physician	Homemaker Services
Skilled Nursing	Chore Services
Physical Therapy	Personal Assistance
Occupational Therapy	Senior Companion
Speech Therapy	Home-Delivered Meals
Medical Social Services	Emergency Response
Nurses Aide Services	Respite Care
Hospice Care at Home	
Pharmacy	
Dietary	
Geriatric Dentistry	
Durable Medical Equipment	

Out-of-Home Services	*Caregivers*
Tax & Legal Assistance	Physicians & Geriatricians
Adult Protective Services	Optometrist & Ophthalmologist
Counseling/Mental Health	Skilled Nurses (LPN, RN, NP)
Adult Day Care	Certified Home Health Aide
Geriatric Day Hospital	Social Worker (BSW, MSW)
Transportation	Dentist
Wellness/Disease Prevention	Therapists (PT, OT, ST)
Respite Care	Pharmacist
Congregate Meals	Audiologist
Hospice Services	Nutritionist
Emergency Response Systems	Companion Volunteer
Telephone Reassurance	Podiatrist
Audiology	Rheumatologist
Podiatry/Beauty Shop	Legal Assistant
Optometry/Ophthalmology	Beautician

LTC Living Arrangements	*LTC Integrated Systems*
Personal Residence	On Lok
Congregate Living	S/HMOs
Assisted Living Centers	CCREs

---

4. living arrangements representing a continuum of living arrangements that provide minor to fairly substantial living assistance service short of nursing home institutionalization; and

5. integrated systems illustrating various delivery systems that combine financing and care delivery, usually including medical and social support services.

General descriptions of the main community-based long-term care services provided by the models represented in this book are described below and are organized within the major service areas.

ASSESSMENT/INFORMATION/REFERRAL-
RELATED SERVICES

These services are listed here first since they are intended to perform general "coordinator" and "gatekeeper" functions and are most often performed at the point of entry of a health care system. They are designed to facilitate a client's referral to the most appropriate available resources. The process of screening and assessing is essential for successful targeting or sorting of the population into categories for proper treatments (Leutz, Abrahams, Greenlick, Kane, & Prottas, 1988).

Client Assessment. Assessment can be viewed as a snapshot of individual functional status and prognosis for future change. Outcome of home care assessment should be a care plan that sustains or improves such functional capability characteristics as affordable, available, appropriate, acceptable, accessible, coordinated, continuous, convenient, dependable, dignified, equitable, family-centered, flexible, professional, safe, secure and timely (Gwyther, 1988).

Case Management. As it pertains to community-based long-term care services, case management is the development and management of an individualized plan of care designed to enable frail and disabled individuals to remain in the community (U.S. Senate, 1988a). Case-management activities include client screening, assessment, care planning, coordination of services to carry out service plans, follow-up, and monitoring. In addition, case managers often provide counseling. An essential feature of this service is the case manager's ongoing responsibility for follow-up. Therefore, case management may also be used to monitor the quality of long-term care services.

When developing community-based home-health care programs, it is essential to define a program's goals before the function of case management can be assigned. For example, if a program goal is to contain costs of community-based care plans, case managers would be expected to estimate the cost of each care plan to increase sensitivity to the costs of the care plans they develop. Or if a program seeks to control nursing home utilization, case managers would be involved in the preadmission screening process. They may also work with nursing home residents for whom it might be possible to return to community living and with hospital discharge planners in targeting patients to community living.

A simultaneous consideration involves defining the target population because the frail elderly will require intense case management, whereas members of a younger, healthier population might be able to serve as their own case managers. Certain subpopulations may require high-intensity case management for a short time or low-intensity management for a longer period to maintain individuals at the highest possible level of functioning and/or delay premature deterioration (Austin & O'Connor, 1989).

Hospital Discharge Planning. The role of discharge planning is to assure that patients receive proper care after they leave the hospital (Williams & Torrens, 1988). Services are performed by a discharge planner and/or a social worker, and, in some cases, other hospital staff may be involved. The discharge planner selects the appropriate services for the patient's posthospital care and explains them to the patient. Discharge planners seldom provide follow-up services to patients once they have left the hospital.

Geriatric Assessment Services. Geriatric assessment or evaluation is a specialized form of discharge planning performed by a multidisciplinary team of professionals with geriatric expertise. The team may include physicians, nurses, social workers, pharmacists, and therapists (Williams & Torrens, 1988). The team assesses the elderly patient's medical, psychological, functional, and social status and recommends a comprehensive plan of treatment and/or care. As with discharge planning, there is no specific follow-up responsibility.

Information and Referral Services. Information and Referral (I&R) services provide the link between individuals and community-based services and is characterized by client self-selection. In 1973, amendments were enacted to the Older Americans Act that made information and referral services for the elderly a priority. Information and referral centers are intended to maintain continuously updated file systems that list community health services, organizations, service providers, and business resources in local areas (Vierck, 1990). I&R workers may also provide counseling and identify gaps in services. I&R services usually do not provide follow-up with clients.

HEALTH AND SUPPORT SERVICES

This category includes a wide variety of services and is presented in two sections: medically related home care and personal and custodial in-home services.

Medically Related Home Care

The first medically related home care service in the United States was modeled after the 1849 Liverpool, England, Nursing Association. Visiting nurse associations of Boston, Buffalo, and Philadelphia have all passed 100th anniversaries (Stanhope, 1989).

Medically related home care includes medically related services and products provided to people requiring medical support in their homes. These services are defined to include primarily the medically related home health care services covered under Medicare and Medicaid.

Physician. The physician plays a key role in quality home care. Often it is the physician who makes the initial referral for home care as a patient returns from a hospital or nursing home, or should a patient's condition change from independence to that requiring assistance with personal care and daily living. It is primarily the physician's responsibility to detail and/or authorize a coordinated plan of care and periodically review the delivery and effectiveness of home care services.

Skilled Nursing. These services are usually provided by a nurse with a graduate degree and involve standard nursing services, education, rehabilitation, and primary case management. Specific duties are differentiated for registered nurses and licensed practical nurses.

Physical Therapy. Normally provided by a licensed physical therapist, these services include assessment, teaching, and exercise and other therapy, as well as assistance with selection of many types of durable medical equipment.

Occupational Therapy. These services are commonly provided by a licensed occupational therapist. They include evaluation of a patient's level of functioning, selection and teaching of activities, and performance of therapy. Occupational therapists also design, fabricate, and fit a wide variety of orthotic devices.

Speech Therapy. Assessment, teaching, and therapy may be provided in the home by a licensed speech therapist. These providers work to minimize the impact of a communication disorder on the client.

Medical Social Services. Mental health services, provided in the home by a licensed social worker, may assist a client in coping with stress, anxiety, or depression. Medical social work is an in-home service, often covered by Medicare. It follows hospitalization and deals with the anxiety and depression often associated with recovery from a serious illness (Reifler & Hansen, 1986).

Nursing Aide Services. These may be provided by licensed practical nurses (LPNs) or homemaker home health aides (HHHAs) and are available under Medicare on an intermittent basis to assist with non-skilled nursing services and personal care.

Hospice Units Within Hospitals. Hospital hospice care is usually provided by an interdisciplinary network of caregivers ranging from physicians and nurses to nurse aides, community volunteers, and, of course, family members. The essential humanism of hospice care can only enhance hospital care while offering patients, families, and staff a system in which one aspect emphasizes cure and the other care. Hospital hospice is often effectively coordinated with home care hospice as patients move between the two systems of care (Wald, Foster, & Wald, 1980).

Hospice Care at Home. A multidisciplinary team, usually hospital based, provides personal and supportive medical care in the home for terminally ill patients and their families. Hospice care is a unique form of community-based service provided to a relatively small client group. Hospice care provides physical, social, and emotional care for the terminally ill and their families. The focus is on pain relief ("quality of death") while allowing the dying person to remain with family and friends. In addition to medical care, hospices provide homemaker, chore, and personal-assistance services.

The health care is generally a team effort that involves all aspects of professional and paraprofessional care. Nurses and home health aides are usually available 24 hours a day, 7 days a week, to make house calls. Medicare pays for both hospital hospice services as well as those available outside the home in freestanding sites or institutionally sponsored settings. Several hospice models exist, ranging from home care to inpatient facilities. Besides the human benefits of hospice,

hospice care at home has been found to be less costly than acute care institutionalization.

Pharmacy. Pharmacists may provide consultative services to home health agencies concerning drugs administered to clients and their possible interactions or side effects. Currently, immunosuppressive drugs are covered by Medicare, as well as IV antibiotic drug therapy at home. Beginning in 1991, Medicare Part B coverage will be extended to all outpatient prescription drugs.

Dietary Needs. Home care providers consult with dietitians regarding diets for patients and their families and suggest appropriate modifications to enable faster recovery and optimal functioning.

Geriatric Dentistry. The essence of geriatric dentistry is knowledge and understanding of the elderly patient in toto, not just the patient's dental needs. The American Society for Geriatric Dentistry, in cooperation with the American Dental Association, works to ensure that ambulatory and institutionalized older people receive excellent dental care.

Optometry/Ophthalmology Services. Eye care is especially important for the elderly; aging eyes require examination, measurement for size and structure, and, often, corrective lenses and surgery.

Audiology Services. Hearing difficulties experienced by the elderly can often be corrected with hearing aids.

Podiatry Services. Foot care is required by the elderly and is especially important for diabetic patients.

Rheumatology Services. Special care for rheumatism-afflicted persons is available.

Durable Medical Equipment. Oxygen equipment, wheelchairs, and walkers are examples of the durable medical equipment that can be provided. These items must be prescribed by a physician in order to be covered by Medicare.

Personal and Custodial In-Home Services

Personal/custodial in-home services are care services of a nontechnical nature, delivered in the client's home. They are often provided by home health aides and supervised by home health nurses, either of whom may also be providers of medically related home care. Other areas of care, such as mental health services, are neither personal/custodial nor medical, but provide necessary support. Some types of care (for example respite and hospice care) may provide personal/custodial, medical, and counseling services. Thus, a separation of health and other support services would be artificial and would not adequately reflect the reality of long-term care. The category of health and support services includes:

Homemaker/Home Health Services. These services are for individuals who do not require medical care but need help with meal preparation and housekeeping (Vierck, 1990). Services are provided by homemaker/home health aides who assist clients with personal care, administration of medications, household work, shopping, cooking, and companionship.

Chore Services. These services provide help in and around the house and include yard work, heavy housecleaning, minor repairs, and errands. They do not include housework, which is a homemaker service.

Personal Assistance. In this group of services, a disabled client is assisted with activities of daily living; for example, eating, dressing, bathing, toileting, mobility, skin care, reading, and translation. In many programs, the personal assistant is referred to as a home health aide or personal care provider who plays the dual role of homemaker/home health aide.

Respite Care. Respite care is intended to give occasional, temporary relief to informal caregivers. The disabled client may receive a combination of homemaker, personal assistance, and chore services. Medicare will cover limited hours of respite care per year for certain beneficiaries. When delivered outside the home, respite care may be provided in a freestanding day care center or with a sponsoring institution, such as a hospital, nursing home, or community agency. Although respite services can be provided outside the home, models providing caregivers a choice of setting reveal preference for in-home services over adult day care or institutional respite.

Advantages to home respite services are low administrative overhead cost, no facility cost, and payment to caregivers only when they are used (Upshur, 1982). Noelker and Bass (1989) suggest that respite can provide the periodic assistance necessary to allow caregivers to continue their primary caregiving roles. Recent research suggests that such interventions as respite care, targeted specifically toward the caregiver, can increase the caregiver's sense of control over his or her environment, reduce burnout, and increase the caregiver's effectiveness (Aronson, Levin, & Lipkowitz, 1984). If such services are available early and regularly, they may avert or postpone the need for more extensive and costly long-term care.

Hospice Care at Home. This care is categorized as both a medically related home service and a personal/custodial service. In addition to the medical care provided, terminally ill clients may require a combination of homemaker, chore, and personal assistance services. Medicare coverage of hospice home care for terminally ill beneficiaries is no longer subject to a maximum number of days of care. Congress is currently considering several provisions to improve hospice coverage.

Senior Companion Program. Created by the Federal Domestic Services Act of 1973, the Senior Companion Program is a key link between professional services and the elderly (Brummell, 1984). This service, which provides regular companionship to the client who may be lonely or isolated, is usually supplied by volunteers, but may include financial or in-kind remuneration.

Volunteer Programs. ACTION is a federal agency that sponsors a number of volunteer programs conducted by the elderly. In addition to the Senior Companion Program described above, the Foster Grandparent Program offers older men and women the opportunity to develop close relationships with children who have special or exceptional needs. Volunteers in this program care for physically, emotionally, and mentally disabled children in institutions and private settings. Participants in the Retired Senior Volunteer Program (RSVP) work in schools, courts, libraries, day care centers, hospitals, and other community services. Regional ACTION offices are located in Atlanta, Boston, Chicago, Dallas, Denver, New York City, Philadelphia, San Francisco, and Seattle.

Home-Delivered Meals. Commonly known as "Meals On Wheels" programs, these services provide nutritionally balanced meals, usually one per day, to elderly clients unable to prepare an adequate meal for themselves. This service is often paid for by Title III of the Older Americans Act.

Emergency Response Systems. These are communication systems that provide a greater sense of well-being and security to disabled or frail clients. Simple services involve daily telephone calls to the client, offering reassurance, and sending assistance if needed. More elaborate services require the use of sophisticated telecommunication devices.

Community-Based Out-of-Home Services

These services are categorized based on their site of provision, and are provided outside the home. Thus, medically related services and personal/custodial services, when provided outside the home, are classified as community-based services.

Adult Protective Services (guardianship or conservatorship). These services provide legal and financial counseling to people unable to manage alone. Protective services can be used for the protection of incapacitated individuals with or without their consent (Vierck, 1990). The majority of states have public guardianship legislation, each with an individual approach to facilitating guardianship for those in danger of harming themselves or who are vulnerable to harm from others (such as family members).

Protective services, which are provided by state or local government agencies, can provide an opportunity for fraud if the chosen guardian is unscrupulous. Adult protection services are often provided by state or local government agencies although there is little funding to implement adult protection laws. Adult protection services are used when an individual is in danger of hurting him or herself. At that point, a guardian is appointed to oversee his/her affairs. This is sometimes used as a remedy for elder abuse. However, adult protective services are most commonly used for older persons with Alzheimer's disease or related disorders.

The National Aging Resource Center on Elder Abuse opened in 1989 with the goal of helping professionals who work with abused adults in regard to information and new developments, research and practice.

Counseling/Mental Health. These services are intended to assist clients in coping with stress, anxiety, depression, or more serious mental health problems. The services may be provided in the community by psychiatrists, psychologists, social workers, clergy, or related mental health professionals. A peer counseling service is often available at the community level, allowing elderly persons to help one another.

Peer Counseling for Older Adults, a self-help approach to mental health, was initiated in the late 1970s. The paraprofessional counseling model reduces the stigma associated with professional mental health services and works to dispel the stereotypes of aging. The concept of counseling benefits both client and counselor in that it helps clients handle their lives better and provides the counselor with a sense of purpose, increased self-esteem, and a chance for personal growth.

Adult Day Care (ADC). Adult day care allows older and disabled persons who would otherwise be in a nursing home to receive care in the community while remaining at home. Most programs provide services for those who do not need 24-hour care but need more care than homemaker services offer. Adult day care covers a wide range of models from intensive programs that closely mirror day hospitals (usually called adult day health care) to social day care programs.

Adult day care involves various types of care, including medically related services (provided in medical day care programs also known as adult day health care programs) and personal/custodial services (provided in some social day care programs); often programs combine these two types of care. Services may be provided in a freestanding center or within a sponsoring institution, such as a hospital, nursing home, or community agency. Adult day care centers provide assistance to clients for parts of each day, usually 5 days a week.

In speaking of ADC, one must be aware of the varying degrees of health services, personal care, and social activities. Aspects of care and tailored care plans for individual clients are the primary considerations that must receive greater attention as ADC expands to serve a wider range of aged and impaired elderly.

Irrespective of models, day care is a financial bargain. Weissert, Cready, and Pawelah (1989) note that a visit from a home health nurse may cost more than $40 for less than an hour, and a 4-hour visit from a homemaker/home health aide may cost over $25. In contrast, a 6-hour day at a typical day care center costs only about $30. The day care center offers periodic health assessment and case management services, a daily meal, and interaction with others (friends, professional caregivers, and helpers). Even on days when clients do not attend day care, they or their at-home companion can call the center for advice and assistance. Day care is labeled as a labor-intensive industry, with labor accounting for over 50% of the cost. Three other major expenses are transportation, facility, and food (Weissert, Cready, & Pawelah, 1989). Day care can also double as respite care for a client's family.

Geriatric Day Hospital Model. This demonstration model is patterned after a component of the British health care system. It offers intensive outpatient care to the frail elderly for whom hospitalization or nursing home placement is otherwise unavoidable. An interdisciplinary geriatrics team provides comprehensive health care without hospitalization whenever possible (Morishita, Siu, Wang, Oken, Cadogan, & Schwartzman, 1989).

Transportation. In most communities, public or private transportation services are available to home care users. This allows them to use other community-based services to perform personal errands, such as shopping. A typical community transportation service offers a volunteer-driven minivan that takes a client to a particular location. Services provided through the Older Americans Act are required to include transportation to and from their programs. Medicaid pays for transportation to and from medical appointments.

Wellness/Disease Prevention Programs. The purpose of these programs is to improve the health status of the older population, increase quality of life, and curtail health expenditures caused by preventable diseases. Health prevention education, nutritional counseling, adult immunization, help with smoking cessation, screening, prevention of fires and accidents, and exercise programs are examples of these services.

Respite Care. This term has been defined above as a personal/custodial in-home service. When delivered outside the home, respite care is considered a community-based service. It may be provided in a freestanding day care center or within a sponsoring institution, such as a hospital, nursing home, or community agency.

Congregate Meals. Like home-delivered meal programs, congregate meal programs provide a nutritionally balanced meal, usually once per day, to participating clients. The meals are served in senior centers, community agencies, or other sponsoring institutions.

Hospice Services. This care for the terminally ill, defined above in both the medical and personal home care sections, is also available outside the home, and in freestanding sites and institutionally sponsored settings.

Emergency Response Systems. These communication systems are often referred to as lifelines. They provide the older or disabled person living at home with a 24-hour link to police or rescue squads and a medical facility. The system works through a transmitter, carried by the user, and a receiver connected to the individual's home. If the user pushes a button on the transmitter, the phone receiver automatically dials an emergency number. The system can also be set so that it will initiate an emergency response if the user has not used the telephone or pushed a designated button for a set period of time.

Telephone Reassurance. This is a community program in which daily telephone calls are made to "check in" with elderly and disabled persons living alone. Telephone reassurance programs typically are staffed by volunteers. In rural areas, mail carriers often provide a similar service.

Legal and Tax Assistance. A service to assist the elderly with confusing legal issues and taxes, including Medicare, Medicaid, and insurance forms, is available.

Barber and Beautician Care. Because looking good is part of feeling good, hair and nail care can also be obtained.

COMMUNITY-BASED LONG-TERM CARE
LIVING ARRANGEMENTS

An appropriate living arrangement is a necessity for the effective use of community-based long-term care services (Sykes, 1988). Residential settings for the elderly and disabled requiring long-term care include facilities providing increasingly greater amounts of outside support and assistance that allow people to "age in place." Although this array of living arrangements suggests a spectrum permitting a smooth transition from totally independent living to increasingly supervised or supportive assistance, analysts of housing options note that people do not tend to move among settings but, more often, age in place as long as possible and then move into medically supervised housing or into a nursing home (Barker, Mitteness, & Wood, 1988).

The dependent elderly live in many different settings. The following were selected as being representative of a possible hierarchy of settings in which the resident's situation ranges from the least to the most dependent.

Personal Residence. In this situation, the dependent client lives at home. This arrangement encompasses ownership or rental of a house, duplex, condominium, apartment, and room in a residential hotel. Support services, emergency response systems, personal care, and family support are often needed by the elderly in order to remain in a personal residence (Vierck, 1990).

Living at home is important to the elderly as an element of independence. In the United States, more than 75% of senior citizens own their own home, resulting in a strong sense of emotional health and security. Such feelings of well-being are often as important to the elderly as the availability of health services (Hereford, 1989).

Congregate Living. This is a group of housing units that is restricted to the elderly and which provides at least one daily shared meal for all residents. Personal and custodial care is usually not provided. Congregate housing was found to be associated with improved survival, reduced unmet needs, reduced institutionalization, and possibly increased hospitalization because of possible better disease detection in congregate housing settings. Congregate housing residents are believed to benefit from increased social involvement, a sense of community, and improved satisfaction with life (Muller, 1989).

Assisted Living Centers. Included in this category are residential care facilities (RCFs), domiciliary care, adult foster care, and board and care facilities. In these settings, personal/custodial care is available. Many of these centers also offer medically related services.

Foster Care. Foster care pioneered as an aftercare service for psychiatric patients and developed with a slim research base (Kane & Kane, 1987). Foster care provides varying degrees of supervision and care for the elderly with moderate degrees of disability. While foster care generally serves the moderately dependent, some programs are placing severely disabled persons in such settings.

A recent study (Kane, Illston, Kane, & Nyman, 1989) comparing Oregon's foster care residents with intermediate care facility residents found minimal differences between the two populations. The sample was profiled as predominantly female, white, widowed, and old (over age 85). Distinctive differences were found in the preference of foster care residents for privacy and the importance of living in a "homelike atmosphere," while the intermediate care facility (ICF) residents valued a more rehabilitative setting. A major conclusion of the study was that foster care has its own place in the continuum-of-care chain and that it is unlikely that foster care can replace the intermediate care facility.

Board and Care. The term "board and care facility" is only one of over 30 terms used throughout the United States to describe domiciliary facilities that provide room, board, laundry service, and varying degrees of protective oversight and nonmedical health and social care for as few as 2 to over 100 residents. Despite the variety of terms, as a result of the Keys Amendment to the Supplemental Security Income, or SSI, program (42 U.S.C. 1382e-e), (P.C. 94-556, Section 505d), all states allow licensing of these types of facilities.

Feder and Scanlon's (1988) review reported that board and care facilities serve a large proportion of chronically mentally ill and other vulnerable groups, a conclusion also reached by the U.S. General Accounting Office (1989). Both reports note that these facilities often do not provide adequate services (such as nursing, specialized therapies, care for the mentally ill, and case management) to meet the needs of residents, who are less likely to receive needed special care than people in their own homes or institutions. Feder and Scanlon conclude that board and care facilities are currently unlikely to substitute for nursing homes because they employ less skilled staff and provide fewer services (due in part to lower payments from public programs), but suggest that they could play a useful role in a long-term care continuum if quality of care and life therein are improved.

The Select Committee on Aging of the U.S. House of Representatives has estimated that there are one million residents of board and care placement and an additional 3.2 million individuals who may be at risk of such placement (McCoy & Conley, personal communication, 1989).

"Aging in Place" Program. A program funded by the Robert Wood Johnson Foundation's "Aging in Place" program is under development by the Colorado Housing and Finance Authority. The goal of the project is to establish models of service delivery that will enable elderly tenants in subsidized housing to remain independent as long as possible. In order to develop efficient, affordable supportive service models, Colorado first conducted a market survey to assess the wants and needs of the elderly residents. Nine congregate living sites have been chosen for such service enhancement as management of care, meals, housekeeping, laundry, personal care, and transportation. Another Aging in Place project, Campus Towers in Chicago, has created a similar program. Eight other state housing and finance authority offices have also established "Aging in Place" programs (Miller, Berg, Bischoff, & Schlenker, 1989).

INTEGRATED SYSTEMS

An integrated system is a model of medical/social health care that integrates financing, management, and care provision. Integrated care systems, with a single payer and broad control over different settings, have organizational incentives that tend to encourage timely use of appropriate levels of care.

Three types of systems that illustrate integrated financing, management, and care provision are discussed below. Each includes case management and uses financial limits to force prioritization of the types of service provided in individual care plans.

On Lok Senior Health Services. Originated in the Chinatown area of San Francisco, this model is directed toward the long-term care needs of a frail, elderly population. An interdisciplinary team provides both case management and health care services. Financing is on a capitated basis (Ansak, 1983).

With the consolidated service system, On Lok works to overcome the fragmentation and discontinuity of health care delivery, whereas single agencies may only provide separate components of care. When clients can no longer attend the day care center, On Lok continues to care for participants, no matter how extensive the care or where it must be provided. No other community-based program in the United States offers all supportive and medical (both acute and chronic) services through the same program, reimbursed by both Medicare and Medicaid capitation payments (Clark, personal communication, 1990).

The capitated approach motivates On Lok to keep its clients well and out of the hospital if possible. Capitation is defined by HCFA as the method of payment for health services in which an individual or institutional provider is paid a fixed per capita amount for each person served with regard to the actual number or nature of services provided to each person.

The average number of hospital days annually per client has fallen steadily since On Lok's inception 18 years ago. For the third quarter of 1987, On Lok's hospitalization rate was 22 days per enrollee per year, slightly lower than the hospitalization rate for the general elderly population. This success rate is commendable since the program serves only the most impaired and chronically ill elderly clients. Only 5% of On Lok clients are in nursing home beds at any one time, although virtually all are assessed to require nursing home level of care. On Lok's costs have run from 8 to 12% lower than traditional care throughout the 1980s (Beresford, 1989). Replication projects are currently being demonstrated. (Refer to chapter 14 for additional information regarding the On Lok program, and to chapter 15 regarding a replication project.)

Social Health Maintenance Organization (S/HMO) Services. Several S/HMOs were funded by the federal government in 1982 as demonstrations to assist the effectiveness of offering a broad range of health, social, and long-term care services to Medicare beneficiaries through an HMO-like (capitated) financing system. The S/HMO concept combines the case management and social support concept with capitated payment.

A major goal of the S/HMO approach to long-term care is to bring the service provider and funding source together under one umbrella. Services generally include the standard medical services offered by HMOs, as well as home health care, homemaker, and chore services. These care-managed systems have grown within Medicare and Medicaid programs but tend to enroll elders with slightly better health status

(Luft & Miller, 1988) and lower current or prior medical and nursing home use (Rossiter & Langwell, 1988) than clients of the traditional fee-for-service system.

There are four sites in the S/HMO demonstration supported by the Health Care Financing Administration and private foundations: Elderplan, Inc., of Brooklyn, New York; Kaiser Permanente Center for Health Research of Portland, Oregon; SCAN Health Plan of Long Beach, California; and Seniors Plus of Minneapolis, Minnesota. The long-term benefit offered by these plans is not intended to cover permanent nursing home placement or extended and very costly community care; rather, participants can receive about $600 to $1,000 per month (depending upon the site) in covered community care services if they are deemed eligible for nursing home care under state guidelines by the site's care management unit. The New York and California sites offer some long-term care benefits to moderately disabled members as well. The Oregon and Minnesota sites included an existing HMO as a sponsor or co-sponsor; the other two are long-term care providers that have developed formal linkages with medical care providers. In either case, the financing approach assures ongoing coordination between acute and long-term care systems (Capitman, 1989a).

Approximately 5% of S/HMO participants meet nursing-home-level-of-care requirements, but there are broad differences across the sites in the proportion of members who access such expanded care benefits as adult day care, paraprofessional home care, durable medical equipment, home modification, medical transportation, and extended skilled treatments and therapies (Leutz, Abrahams, Greenlick, Kane, & Prottas, 1988). These differences are due to variations in targeting criteria and care management practices (Abrahams, Capitman, Leutz, & Macho, 1988).

Continuing Care Retirement Communities (CCRCs). CCRCs combine financing and delivery of long-term care services and provide some form of catastrophic insurance for noncovered services. Residents pay a monthly charge. Housing, social and recreational services, and medical and preventive services are provided on the community's "campus." Also included may be annual physicals, emergency response systems, therapies, hospitalization coverage, prescriptions, and social services.

This model is primarily accessible to the most affluent elders since entrance and maintenance fees are high.

A 1987 survey by the American Association of Homes for the Aging found that one third of all CCRCs were providing "extensive" health benefits (Cohen, Tell, Batten, & Larson, 1988). The three levels of benefits from CCRCs described by Cohen et al. were based on their coverage of nursing home expenses. Type A programs cover lifetime use of nursing home services financed by pooled entrance and monthly fees. Residents of these communities are not charged extra for nursing home services. Type B programs place a ceiling on the amount of nursing home services each resident may receive. Services beyond that amount are charged to the resident on a fee-for-service basis. The third variation, Type C, charges for all nursing home services on a fee-for-service basis.

A CCRC resident may move from congregate housing, through assisted living, and then to nursing home care without moving from the campus. To join such a community requires the payment of an entrance fee and monthly charge. In 1986, 7,000 CCRCs provided retirement living and health care to over 100,000 elderly Americans.

The reasons for joining CCRCs include ready access to services and protection for spouse (Cohen et al., 1988). Another noteworthy development is the expansion of the CCRC model to cover people who live in their own homes. This Life Care At Home (LCAH) model provides all of the nonhousing services of a CCRC and is also financed by entry and monthly fees (Tell, Cohen, & Wallack, 1987).

Conclusions Regarding Integrated Systems. Integrated financing and delivery systems are currently in evaluation; while they show promise, they have critical issues to consider. The three types of systems discussed here attempt to integrate financing, management, and care provision. Each uses financial limitation to force prioritization of the types of service in individual care plans. These are combined with case management consistent with the episodic clinical pattern of care associated with heavy users of service.

The On Lok model is limited to some degree by its dependence upon a cohesive community structure. One concern with the S/HMO model is the possible incentive for underutilization of services. A major criticism of the CCRC model is related to access: High entry and maintenance fees make it an option only for the most financially stable elderly. While each of these two models has its weakness, these models have each met with success in providing better coordination of care than traditional models.

The fragmented nature of the traditional system produces transfer costs that limit a patient's movement between levels of care. Integrated care systems, with a single payer and broad control over different settings, have organizational incentives that tend to encourage timely use of appropriate levels of care.

2

Payers

Community-based services are financed by a variety of federal, state, and local public programs; limited private insurance; out-of-pocket payments; and donated funds and services of family and friends. Spending for community-based long-term care services was estimated by the Congressional Budget Office to be $9.1 billion for home health care in 1985. Direct out-of-pocket payments covered $3.7 billion, or 40% of this amount. Private long-term care insurance paid for 4% (U.S. Senate, 1989). Several of the major financing sources are summarized below.

MEDICARE

Medicare, Title XVIII of the Social Security Act, is a federal health insurance program for individuals aged 65 and over and certain disabled persons. Operated through the Health Care Financing Administration of the United States Department of Health and Human Services, it is administered locally through private insurance carriers. Medicare is divided into two distinct and separately financed parts. Part A, which covers hospital insurance, is available to anyone 65 or older who has enough quarters of coverage employment to qualify for Social Security. Most enrollees' spouses, if they are 65, are also eligible. There are special requirements disabled individuals must meet in order to qualify for Medicare; others age 65 or older may purchase coverage. Part A benefits are paid for from a portion of the payroll tax on workers. Part B covers physician services, outpatient hospital care, and lab services. Individuals who qualify for Part A must "opt out" of Part B if they do not want its coverage. Enrollees who participate in Part B must pay a monthly premium of $28.60, an amount that is usually deducted from a recipient's monthly Social Security check. The benefits for both Parts A and B are described below.

Part A

Part A of Medicare, Hospital Insurance, helps pay for inpatient hospital care, some inpatient care in a skilled nursing facility, home health care, and hospice care. However, Medicare will fully cover only the first 60 days of hospitalization after a patient pays a $592 deductible for each spell of illness. The patient pays $148 per day in coinsurance for days 61 to 90. Beneficiaries are liable to share costs (known as coinsurance charges) with the government in the amount of $296 per day for lifetime reserve days. After the reserve days are used up, the patient or his or her insurer pays the entire bill.

Regarding nursing home care, an enrollee must be hospitalized for at least 3 days prior to entering a skilled nursing facility care in order for Medicare to help pay for the cost of nursing home services. For each spell of illness, Medicare will pay for all covered services for the first 20 days. For days 21 to 100, the patient is required to pay $74 per day in coinsurance; after which the patient picks up the entire tab.

For home health care, Medicare covers up to 21 consecutive days for enrollees needing full-time care, or up to 35 hours per week for those who need skilled care for a period of less than 4 days per week. The beneficiary must be homebound, and services must be ordered and reviewed regularly by a doctor.

Medicare covers up to 210 days of hospice care. It is predicted that Medicare Part A, which is funded by payroll taxes, will begin to outspend incoming revenues by 1995 and be totally exhausted by 2002 (Kron, Iverson, & Pastor, 1989).

Part B

Part B, Medical Insurance, helps pay for medically necessary doctor's services, outpatient hospital services, home health care, and other medical services and supplies. Both parts A and B entail premiums, deductibles, and coinsurance payments.

Other Medicare Information

Although Medicare represents the largest single source of public financing for home health care, such services were designed primarily as short-term postacute benefits. After a beneficiary meets an annual $75 deductible, Medicare pays 80% of what it determines is the reasonable charge for doctor and other services. The beneficiary is responsible for the remaining 20% and any amount that exceeds Medicare's approved charge. Medicare pays only for prescription drugs administered in the hospital and for immunosuppressive drugs.

Medicare is intended to pay for acute medical care for people 65 years or older, but it pays only for skilled nursing care, whether in a nursing home or at home. Medicare does not cover custodial care (help with bathing or eating) unless such care is provided concurrently with skilled care.

MEDICAID

Medicaid, Title XIX of the Social Security Act, was enacted to assist low-income persons with medical expenses. Medicaid primarily provides reimbursement for care for eligible individuals in nursing homes. Medicaid services include home health and personal care, home- and community-based (waiver) services, and related other services. Medicaid home health care is defined in federal regulations as nursing services, home health aide services, and medical supplies and equipment. Speech, physical, and occupational therapy may be offered at the state's option.

Personal Care. Personal care is an optional Medicaid benefit that a few states (notably Massachusetts, New York, Oklahoma, Oregon, and Texas) have used extensively. Such services generally are intended to accommodate long-term chronic or maintenance home care rather than the short-term acute care generally provided through home health services. Included are nonmedical but medically oriented services to assist persons with physical dependency needs in activities in daily living (HCFA, Medical Assistance Manual 5-140-00).

Home- and Community-Based Services (HCBS). Home- and community-based services were first extended as a Medicaid benefit in 1981 by the Omnibus Budget Reconciliation Act (PL 97-35, Section 2176), which authorized a new type of Medicaid waiver, commonly referred to as a "Medicaid 2176 waiver." By early 1983, 34 states had applied for Medicaid 2176 waivers (Eustis, Greenberg, & Patton, 1984).

HCBS are available to those at risk of institutionalization in a hospital or nursing home, and can be provided under 2176 waivers, which permit states to cover populations and provide services (particularly in-home supportive rather than medically or nursing-oriented care) not generally financed by Medicaid. Services that states may cover include case management, homemaker, home health aide, personal care, adult day health care, habilitation, respite care, and other services approved by the state Medicaid agency and HCFA as cost effective.

According to Lipson (1988), about 30 states offer case management, personal care, and homemaker services under HCBS, while about 20 states offer family respite and adult day care to their elderly populations. Additional, but rarely offered, services are foster care, transportation, and home adaptations.

Other Medicaid community-based long-term health care services include private-duty nursing, case management, and therapies. Private-duty nursing is an optional Medicaid service provided by some states. Case management (which had not been available under waivers since 1981) was authorized as a separate Medicaid optional service in 1986. Specialized therapies represent optional Medicaid services that can be provided in the community to enhance the recipient's ability to remain independent. Medicaid covers physical therapy, occupational therapy, and services for individuals with speech, hearing, and language disorders if they are prescribed by a physician and provided by registered or certified professionals.

Waivers. To obtain waivers, states must demonstrate that they will safeguard recipient health and welfare, provide audited financial statements, evaluate each recipient's initial and continuing need for institutional-level services, permit recipients a choice of institutional and noninstitutional services, and provide reports on quality, access, and cost effectiveness to HCFA. Waivers were originally authorized for 3 years and are to be extended for additional 5-year periods unless states have failed to meet the waiver conditions (42 C.F.R. 441.304).

Medicaid Shortcomings. Because Medicaid is a joint federal-state program, it lacks national uniformity. Each state operates with different rules, eligibility requirements, schedules of benefits, and administrative structures. Therefore, persons in identical circumstances may receive Medicaid benefits in one state but not in another (U.S. Senate, 1986).

Medicaid currently fails to provide coverage for almost two-thirds of the poor elderly (U.S. House of Representatives, 1986).

Aside from ethical issues of not meeting the basic needs of the elderly population, inadequate care leads to increased costs. Without proper care elderly people cannot practice preventive medicine and do not receive prompt treatment. Consequences are higher costs and longer term treatments for these unfortunate individuals (Kron, Iverson, & Pastor, 1989).

With this news, it is expected that Medicaid services will soon be carefully rationed. In fact, Oregon may be the trailblazer by becoming the first state in the union to implement a full-scale system of health-care rationing for Medicaid patients. Oregon State Senate President John Kitzhabaer, a physician, has presented a plan that seeks to place, in order of priority, every medical procedure performed, its cost, and— perhaps most noteworthy—its likelihood of producing more "well years" of life. For example, prenatal care may take precedence over a liver transplant for a confirmed 65-year-old alcoholic (Gaffney, 1990).

THE SOCIAL SERVICES BLOCK GRANT

In 1981, Title XX of the Social Security Act was restructured into the Social Services Block Grant (SSBG). The major purpose of the SSBG is to prevent or reduce inappropriate institutional care by providing for community-based care. Through the SSBG, all 50 states provide a number of community-based long-term care services for a broad range of needy individuals, including children, the disabled, and the elderly. Services typically included under SSBG are personal care and home-maker services, case management, adult day care, and home-delivered meals. Unfortunately, SSBG services are not readily available in many communities due to competing demands and limited funding. SSBG funds are distributed to states according to state population, and the state has considerable flexibility in using its funds. There is no require-ment for a state to match funds or to impose income eligibility services, payment, or quality assurance. Title XX, like Medicaid regulations and eligibility requirements, varies from state to state; since funds are limited, the program can only provide services to a limited number of persons (Rabin & Stockton, 1987).

THE OLDER AMERICANS ACT

The Older Americans Act was adopted in 1965 and reenacted in 1987 to improve the emotional, physical, economic, social, civic, cultural, and recreational well-being of the nation's elderly, defined as persons age 60 or over. The program was developed by the Administration on Aging (AOA), an agency of the Department of Health and Human Services.

State Units on Aging. A national network known as the National Association of State Units on Aging (NASUA), has been created to coordinate community services for older people. The grassroots level of the network is organized into Area Agencies on Aging under the National Association of Area Agencies on Aging. This organization is funded by the Administration on Aging of the Department of Health and Human Services and by membership dues; it serves as a public interest group that provides information, technical assistance, and professional development support to State Units on Aging.

Title III Services. Title III of the Older Americans Act finances comprehensive, coordinated services in several categories. The purpose of Title III, which authorizes grants to states for services to older persons, is to foster the development of a comprehensive and coordinated service system for older persons in order to:

1. secure and maintain maximum independence and dignity in a home environment for older persons capable of self-care;
2. remove individual and social barriers to economic and personal independence for older persons; and
3. provide a continuum of care for the vulnerable elderly. Services funded under the act include case management, preinstitutional screening, homemaker, home health aide, home-delivered meals, adult day care, shopping, transportation, legal services, counseling, and information/referral services. Of these services, the following have been given priority by Congress (U.S. Senate, 1988a): access services (transportation, outreach, information and referral), legal assistance, and in-home services.

The Older Americans Act Amendments of 1986 created a new service program of nonmedical in-home services for the frail elderly. Frail individuals are defined as those with physical or mental disabilities that restrict their ability to perform daily tasks or threaten their capacity to live independently. While in-home services have been a priority since 1975, no separate authorization was made under prior law.

Title III-D. This in-home provision authorizes payment for home-maker and home health aide services, visiting and telephone reassurance, chore maintenance, in-home respite care, adult day care as respite for families, and minor modification of homes in an amount not to exceed $150 per client. Under Title III, grants are made to state Agencies on Aging, which in turn award funds to 670 area agencies in order to plan, coordinate, and advocate a comprehensive service system for older persons. States are required to match their federal grants by contributing 15% in private or public nonfederal funds.

Eligibility. The Older Americans Act imposes no income eligibility requirements, although the OAA programs are targeted at low-income (below poverty), minority, severely disabled, and isolated elderly. Title III programs are often used for persons not meeting Medicaid eligibility criteria. However, its impact is limited due to the lack of adequate funds.

THE VETERANS ADMINISTRATION

In addition to the public programs described above, the Veterans Administration (VA) provides long-term care services in a variety of noninstitutional settings. Programs include community residential care, hospital-based home care, and adult care (U.S. Senate, 1988b). Under the VA's community residential care program, disabled or elderly veterans who are unable to live independently are provided limited personal care and supervision in a private home. In 1966, 11,600 veterans participated in the program.

Home Care Program. The VA's hospital-based home care program is designed to enable chronically ill veterans to leave a hospital setting earlier than would otherwise be possible by making health care available in the home. Under the guidance of a multidisciplinary team, the veteran's family is trained to meet his or her individual needs. The VA's adult day care program, providing primarily medical services, has grown slowly since authorization in 1983, and, by 1986, had 12,138 veterans enrolled.

In 1985, the VA served approximately 1.3 million veterans at a cost of $8 billion. During that year, the VA provided approximately $800 million for nursing home care and $600 million for home health care. In 1984, there were approximately 4 million veterans over age 65 who were eligible for nursing home care, a figure that will increase to approximately 7.2 million in 1990 and 9 million by the year 2000. By 2010, half of all men over 65 will be veterans; however, by 2020 figures will drop to slightly less than one-third (U.S. House of Representatives, 1986).

A major limitation to the VA program is that it is not coordinated with other major health and long-term care programs such as Medicare and Medicaid; this lack of coordination increases the inefficient allocation of resources and beneficiary confusion.

HOUSING-RELATED PUBLIC PROGRAMS

Federal Loans. The Housing Act of 1959 created Section 202 to provide direct federal loans to nonprofit private organizations for the construction of housing for the elderly and disabled. Participating residents must be capable of independent living and must be either over age 62 or be developmentally disabled/handicapped and aged 18 to 62. The Housing and Community Development Act of 1987 combined low-interest loans with an initial operating cost subsidy. Sponsors of Section 202 projects are expected to provide services for independent living, most of which are funded by Title III, the Older Americans Act, or SSBGs (Rechkovsky, 1989).

Congregate Housing Services Program. The Housing and Community Development Act of 1978 created the Congregate Housing Services Program (CHSP) as a demonstration program to provide nonmedical services to vulnerable elderly and handicapped Section 202 residents. The Housing and Community Development Act of 1987 expanded CHSP. The program was implemented where community supportive services were inadequate but was limited to 66 project sites. The costs of services are shared by the recipients, with payments based on a sliding scale. Professional Assessment Committees (PACs) are required to evaluate individuals to determine services to be provided, and to recommend a higher level of care when necessary (Rechkovsky, 1989).

Federal Housing Administration (FHA) Mortgage Insurance. Section 232 of the National Housing Act was amended through the Housing and Urban-Rural Recovery Act of 1983 to provide FHA mortgage insurance for nursing homes, intermediate care activities, and board and care homes. Insurance is available for new construction, substantial rehabilitation, and for the installation of fire safety equipment. To be eligible, board and care homes must serve older adults and must have five or more bedrooms. Both proprietary and private nonprofit organizations are eligible for these federally insured mortgages (Rechkovsky, 1989).

Mortgage Coinsurance. In December 1987, the Department of Housing and Urban Development (HUD) published a proposed rule that would establish a new mortgage coinsurance program under Section 232, covering new construction or substantial rehabilitation of board and care homes. The availability of coinsurance should substantially reduce the amount of time required to process Section 232 loans.

Rent Subsidy. Another recent HUD amendment to the Section 8 rent subsidy program allows Section 8 subsidies to be used for shared housing arrangements, including board and care homes (Dobkin, 1989). FHA mortgage insurance is available also for elderly rental housing projects under Section 231 and Section 221(d)(3),(4).

Community Development Block Grants (CDBGs). CDBGs provide relatively unrestricted grants to cities for activities assigned to assist low/moderate-income persons, eliminate slums and blight, and help meet urgent community development needs. The CDBG program has been used to support board and care homes and other long-term care facilities as well as supportive services.

Supplemental Security Income (SSI). The primary federal support for board and care facilities is the Supplemental Security Income program created by the 1972 amendments to the Social Security Act. The purpose of the program is to institute uniform national eligibility and payment standards for redistributing income to poor persons who are also aged, disabled, or blind.

The SSI program was created as a bottom level for funding support with the expectation that states would supplement the basic federal payments. Most states participate in this program through State Supplemental Payment (SSP) programs. SSI/SSP programs are the primary payers for board and care and serve as an income transfer rather than a vendor payment program (Capitman, 1989b). Many board and care residents receive at least the basic SSI payment of $354 a month, while 43 states provide an additional state supplement for needy board-and-care residents (Dobkin, 1989).

Home Equity Conversion. Community-based care for the elderly can also be funded through home equity conversion, which permits aged homeowners to convert part of their equity to cash, without having to give up their homes. In 1987, a demonstration program on home equity conversion mortgages for the elderly was undertaken through the Housing and Community Development Act. In the program, the Department of Housing and Urban Development and the Administration on Aging will jointly provide counseling services to assist prospective borrowers in selecting a mortgage. The Federal National Mortgage Association and the Federal Home Loan Mortgage Corporation also are participating in the program.

SUPPORTIVE SERVICES
FOR SENIOR HOUSING

Aging In Place. Demonstration projects exploring the "aging in place" phenomena are currently in progress at 10 sites. State Housing and Finance Authorities are developing additional ways to finance housing for the elderly. Upon implementation, the program will be evaluated, with an eye toward nationwide replication. The goal of the program is to establish models of service delivery that will enable elderly tenants in subsidized housing to remain independent.

In order to develop efficient, affordable, supportive service models, each site conducted a market survey to assess the needs of the elderly residents before proceeding to develop in-house programs. Typical services offered by these programs are care management, meals, housekeeping, laundry, personal care, and transportation.

PUBLIC PROGRAMS

A variety of other public programs also finance home- and community-based health and social services. These include the Indian Health Service and the Civilian Health and Medical Program for the Uniformed Services (CHAMPUS). In addition, most states fund some community-based long-term care programs through general revenues. Other federal block grant programs make funds available to states that may be used for community-based long-term care. These include Alcohol/Drug

Abuse and Mental Health Block Grants and Energy Assistance Block Grants.

PRIVATE SOURCES OF FUNDING

Private Insurance. Private insurance is limited in the long-term care area; and Medicare supplemental insurance does not cover long-term care. Private long-term care insurance, which covers care in a nursing home and sometimes home health care, plays a minimal role in financing community-based care. However, several life insurance firms offer a long-term care rider attached to a life insurance policy that pays for nursing home care, intermediate care, and home care. These programs have been approved by 12 states (*Mature Market Report,* 1988). Several recent reports (e.g., Rivlin & Wiener, 1988; Shearer, 1989) have been critical of the ability of these policies to provide adequate long-term care coverage for seniors.

Only the more affluent elders are financially able to purchase long-term care insurance, and most of these plans have been criticized for high costs, low loss ratios, and restrictive or under-developed enrollment and underwriting criteria (Firman, 1988). The Department of Health and Human Services (Sullivan, 1989) reported that more than 37 million Americans lack health insurance and more than 11 million of them make less than $10,000 per year. Sullivan suggests that federal, state, and local governments; insurance companies; and nonprofit groups must work together to find ways to pay for long-term health care.

The challenge for insurers is to provide consumers with financial protection, broader coverage for home- and community-based care, and timely access to quality services. Simultaneously, insurers need to manage risk effectively to keep insurance affordable. As insurance companies expand to these broader, more accessible benefits for home- and community-based services, two things are expected to occur. First, the loosely defined and/or not widely regulated services will become standardized. Second, organizations with high-quality long-term care assessment and case management programs will be invaluable in providing long-term care risk-management services to insurers. The basic risk-management features of a fiscally viable and clinically meaningful long-term care insurance policy are accurate assessment of the factors that predict the potential use of and actual need for long-term care; mechanisms for cost containment and quality assurance through service planning based on assessment of need; coordination of services and resources; monitoring of service provider performance; and regular updating of the client's actual functional status and need for service (Lyons, 1989b).

Case Managed Insurance Benefits. The American Association of Homes for the Aging (AAHA) has sponsored a long-term care insurance program for its member retirement communities. AAHA spent almost two years researching the long-term care insurance needs of its members, developed prototype policies based on these needs, and then entered an agreement with a high-quality insurance carrier to underwrite the program. The insurance company, UNUM, developed a service delivery agreement with a nationwide LTC case management network, The Family Caring Network, so that the program is now a collaborative effort between the AAHA, the insurance company, and a provider organization. Dozens of hospitals, HMOs, and religious/fraternal organizations are exploring similar relationships with carriers and providers both at local/regional and national levels (Lyons, 1989b).

New Insurance Trends. Nearly 200,000 long-term care insurance policies were purchased in the first six months of 1989, bringing the total sold to 1.3 million. In December 1988, 103 companies offered such policies, and six companies joined the ranks in 1989. Nearly 90% of long-term care insurance policies have been sold to individuals, 8% through group associations, 3% were employer-sponsored, and less than 1% were sold as life insurance policy riders. More employers are offering or will be offering long-term care insurance policies (*LTC Management,* 1989a).

Model Insurance Project. The Robert Wood Johnson Foundation is currently working with eight states to develop long-term care insurance. The project has conducted surveys to determine long-term care service needs, to gather data on projected expenditures, and to design a model of home- and community-based care with the cooperation of government officials and private-sector individuals (Schlenker, Miller, Berg, Bischoff, & Butler, 1989).

Private Charities. United Way agencies and other private charities also account for the several million dollars that have been spent on home health care for the elderly and disabled population. Funding is dispersed through grants to selected service agencies. Numerous community-based care projects are funded by foundations and other organizations, such as the Kellogg Foundation, the Robert Wood Johnson Foundation, the PEW Memorial Trust, and others. Most service agencies hold special events and fundraisers and apply for grants to meet approximately 40% of the budget.

Continuing Care Retirement Community. Another private financing source is the evolving continuing care retirement community, or life care community. These residential communities provide housing, meals, housekeeping, social activities, and congregate meals for an entrance and monthly fee.

Family Care. As mentioned earlier, most custodial care is provided informally, primarily through the unpaid assistance of family and friends. This assistance often keeps the chronically ill and disabled who do not need acute medical care out of institutions.

Most community-based long-term care programs have creatively coordinated several funding sources to consolidate a fragmented financing system and centralize service delivery. The funding infrastructures for 16 states are listed in chapter three, and are fully described for each of the 12 models presented in the second section of this book.

3

Licensure and Certification

A broad array of public and private sector quality assurance programs exists for community-based long-term care services. It is generally agreed that a quality assurance program must have three components: standards that define and measure the attributes of quality to be regulated, a monitoring procedure to determine whether practice conforms with those standards, and a means of enforcement to discipline violators, achieve correction, and deter future misconduct (Institute of Medicine, 1986). The licensure for home health agencies and board and care facilities will be described below, followed by a discussion of the quality assurance regulations of major public payment programs and regulations of private sector programs.

PUBLIC SECTOR REGULATION OF COMMUNITY-BASED HEALTH CARE: STATE

State Licensure of Home Health Agencies

Currently, 40 states license home health agencies that provide nursing, home health aide, homemaker, and other related services, but it is predicted that by the end of 1990 all states will have a licensure option. Many states were encouraged to adopt home health licensing laws after Medicare was enacted in 1965. Until 1980, Medicare would reimburse only those proprietary agencies that were licensed by a state. Perhaps for this reason, most states define home health agencies similar to the definition ascribed to by Medicare; that is, an organization providing part-time or intermittent skilled nursing services and at least one therapeutic service (Johnson, 1988; American Bar Association, 1984).

Thus agencies operating in these states and providing only a single service, such as home nursing, need not be licensed at all. Licensing standards are primarily structural and rarely exceed Medicare standards (described below). However, there is an extensive national movement for state legislatures to pass licensure and training requirements for home health aides.

There is little information about the experience of state home care licensing agencies. Little is published about the types of violations found, frequency of repeat violations, and enforcement actions and their efforts. Harrington and Grant's (1988) study of home health care regulation (a combination of licensure and certification) in California revealed that California's licensing standard regarding staff qualifications, training, and experience exceed those under Medicare. A 37-state survey by the American Association of Retired Persons produced similar findings (Riley, 1989). A 6-state survey of long-term reform reported by Justice, Ethredge, Luehrs, and Burwell (1989), describes the level of development of their community-based service systems and quality assurance structures.

Quality Assurance Systems for 16 States. A 16-state survey was conducted by Miller et al. (1989) for a study funded by the Health Care Financing Administration (HCFA) as part of its response to congressional mandates contained in the Medicare Catastrophic Coverage Act of 1988 (P.L. 100-360). The survey was designed to gather information regarding quality assurance mechanisms being implemented for long-term care services in community-based and custodial settings.

A brief overview of the efforts on the part of these 16 states is presented to show the reader that some impressive efforts are in progress to assure quality community-based care. The reader will also notice a strategically designed infrastructure that each state has created to consolidate services and funding to provide a more efficient, cost-effective delivery system.

ARIZONA—Arizona has not adopted traditional Medicaid and was granted a freedom-of-choice waiver from the Health Care Financing Administration to implement the Health Care Organization (HCO) demonstration program called AHCCCS (Arizona Health Care Cost Containment System). Started in 1982, the program was designed to provide acute and long-term care to the poor. Home care became a part of the service system in October 1988 when its provision was contracted by county programs via a competitive bidding process. Clients are supervised by case managers who assess clients and develop care plans.

Arizona's AHCCCS has established a set of standards for case managers that includes requirements for quarterly client contact, written service plans, service authorization, and medical record reviews. Case managers assess all clients, develop care plans, and monitor and follow clients. All service providers are Medicaid certified, a process that involves an additional level of monitoring by the state certification agency.

ARKANSAS—The Arkansas Department of Human Services is the umbrella agency for the Division of Economic and Medical Services and the Division of Aging and Adult Services. The Arkansas State Unit of Aging has recently applied for a Medicaid waiver. In preparation, the division has designed significant system changes in the planning and utilization of long-term care services.

Arkansas' new long-term care plan, Project 2000, encompasses private sector development of residential care facilities, feasibility studies on LTC insurance and S/HMOs, and volunteer-led coalitions as key participants in the development and implementation of long-term care. Quality assurance and data information sets are components of the program. The project is funded by an Administration on Aging grant, and has added case management training as a monitoring vehicle for the quality assurance plan.

COLORADO—The Colorado Department of Social Services has recently drafted a long-term care plan. The effort was launched in consideration of the increasing elderly and disabled population in Colorado and projections that the number of persons in need of long-term health care is expected to more than double between the years 1980 and 2000. Additionally, Colorado has found that long-term care provided in home and community settings is preferred by clients and is frequently more cost effective than nursing home care.

Colorado has developed a single point of entry for clients seeking services; a consolidation of funding and human resources; standardization of terms, services, and quality of care definitions; a case-mix reimbursement approach to nursing home services; certification and training for home health services and professional personnel; and legislation to assist the process of implementing these infrastructural changes.

FLORIDA—Florida has the highest percentage of residents over the age of 65 in the United States. Its fastest growing population segment is the 85-and-over age group. The first priority of Florida's Department of Health and Rehabilitative Services is to deal with the lack of service and limited funding for service expansion. The Better Living for Seniors initiative is an effort to keep older Floridians independent, in good health, and in their own homes whenever possible by providing quality services. Service coordination is intended to centralize access to services with ongoing efforts for improvement of the programs.

Florida's Aging and Adult Services program implemented an Administration on Aging grant entitled "Targeted Innovative Strategies for Assessing Quality of In-Home Services to the Elderly." The program addressed the need for improved methods of determining client satisfaction with in-home services to the elderly. Specific services were homemaker, home-delivered meals, and personal care services provided to frail, homebound elderly.

ILLINOIS—The Illinois Department of Aging (IDoA) became a state-cabinet-level agency in 1973. The Department's mission is to provide maximum independence, health, dignity, and quality of life for older persons through the development, implementation, and administration of a substate service delivery system. The Department's Division of Administrative Compliance monitors the entities comprising this service delivery system and that encompass all service contracts: the Area Agencies on Aging, Case Coordination Units, and Community Care Program (CCP) vendor agencies. The CCP's dramatic growth led to increased vendor competition for service contracts and subsequent low bids, thereby threatening program quality. In 1985, Illinois Governor James Thompson appointed a Procurement Task Force to work with IDoA to address the issue of cost versus quality, resulting in the current Quality Assurance Program. Fiscal Year 1987 saw the implementation of the Quality Assurance Program's first objective with the compliance monitoring of 100% of Community Care Program vendors and case coordination units.

MAINE—The Bureau of Maine's Elderly consolidated to include the Division of Adult Services in late 1989. The new agency, The Bureau of Aging and Adult Service, is designed to better coordinate services to vulnerable adults by combining services within a single bureau of the Department of Human Services. The program incorporates funding from both state and federal sources, such as Title III and Medicaid

Waiver 2176, to create a comprehensive range of services that include living-quarter adaptation and medical equipment.

MARYLAND—A current effort of the Maryland Office on Aging is to coordinate funding and services for long-term care in order to eliminate the problem of fragmentation and competing demands for services. The state is combining all state and federal funds and creating a single point of entry, with services being managed by the local Area Agency on Aging. A statewide consortium has developed service standards for the quality of in-home services to be adopted as state law.

MINNESOTA—In 1985, the Minnesota Department of Human Services (DHS) was granted a Home and Community-Based Model Waiver for Chronically Ill Children. In 1987, the Waiver was amended to be a Home and Community-Based Model Waiver for Chronically Ill Individuals of Age 65 who need hospital-level care. A Community Alternative Care Program was developed to provide safe home care in the community for individuals who would otherwise need to live in an acute care hospital, spend an extraordinary amount of time in a hospital, or need frequent hospitalization.

Additionally, Minnesota's DHS has a Preadmission Screening/Alternative Care Grant Program designed to prevent or delay nursing home care for the elderly. The evaluation team includes a social worker and a public health nurse, and could include the client's personal physician. The team then recommends an appropriate setting (nursing home, patient's home, or alternate housing) and develops a plan to provide needed services. Alternative Care Grants (ACG) are available to help pay for such community services, foster care, personal care, and case management. For ACG units, the cost of care cannot be greater than the average monthly cost of nursing home care.

A Minnesota care model that has successfully combined the components of service and funding is The Block Nurse Program. (It is fully described in chapter 6. Generations Assisted Living, another Minnesota program that has created a successful service and financial infrastructure, is fully described in chapter 12.)

NEW YORK—Over a decade old, New York's Long-Term Care Program (also known as the Nursing Home Without Walls) provides and coordinates the delivery of comprehensive services to the chronically ill and disabled so that they may be cared for at home. The Nursing Home Without Walls Program has been replicated by the states of Hawaii and Rhode Island and is currently being considered by other states as a model for community-based long-term care. The Nursing Home Without Walls model is presented in chapter 10.

New York's Expanded In-Home Services for the Elderly Program (EISEP), enacted in 1986, is funded at a ratio of 75 state dollars: 25 local dollars. Funding is administered through area agencies on aging to provide expanded nonmedical in-home support services, case management, respite care, and ancillary services for functionally impaired elderly. The New York State Office for the Aging has designed a model system for assuring the quality of in-home services administered by the New York State Office on Aging, the New York Department of Health, and the State Department of Human Services. Its basic premise is a consistency in quality care standards to be used by all providers and in client outcome measures that can be applied differentially to clients, depending on their functional impairment and the nature of the service and case management required.

This model will apply to the entire New York home health delivery system, with the potential for replication by other states. It is believed that the greatest attribute of the program will be the move from a retrospective to a prospective "occurrence" approach, thus creating a quality assurance system that addresses quality issues as a client is entering the care system as opposed to when exiting the system.

OHIO—Ensuring the quality of community-based long-term care has been addressed by Ohio's State Department of Human Services in a program called PASSPORT. Started in 1984, the purpose of PASSPORT is to expand community-based long-term care; adult day care; home-delivered meals; home health aide and homemaker services; skilled nursing; physical, occupational, and speech therapies; medical equipment; and long-term care case management. The PASSPORT system of care is presented in chapter 9.

OREGON—Project Independence was established in 1975 by the Oregon state legislature to assure in-home services to the elderly who wish to live at home. In 1980, Oregon instituted a statewide preadmission screening activity which, under state supervision, is carried out by local area agencies on aging. In 1981, all long-term care and Office of Aging Administration programs were combined into the Senior Services Division. That same year, Oregon received the first Home- and Community-Based Service Waiver. In 1982, the Senior Services Division initiated a relocation of nursing facility residents to a less restrictive living situation, with needs for living planned for and secured at the community level.

The in-home services provided by Project Independence were expanded through community-based social services. Alternative Community Care was formed for the following services: home care, personal care, homemaker, assisted living, adult foster homes, residential care facilities, and specialized living facilities. A successful Oregon Assisted Living program is presented in chapter 13.

SOUTH CAROLINA—The South Carolina Health and Human Services Finance Commission appears to be one of the forerunners in developing and implementing a statewide quality assurance system that encompasses all human service programs. A unique feature of the state's community-based home care program is the concept of combining several services into a single service with levels of care within it. Many discrete quality assurance activities interrelate to form a systematic, comprehensive whole that reaches beyond the easily identified components of quality assurance into nearly all aspects of service management. The quality assurance system allows collaborative effort rather than competitive action and involves the entire service enterprise. It is based on enhancement rather than control and, like the system in New York, is proactive rather than reactive.

TENNESSEE—Besides the standard Medicaid Quality Review regulations and Joint Commission on Accreditation of Healthcare Organizations Certification, the Tennessee Department of Human Services has created a Statement of Care Committee to cover skilled nursing, infusion, and other high-technology home care. There is concern that quality assurance be built into the service program so that the system is not overpowered by paperwork.

The Tennessee Commission on Aging developed a model for a quality assurance system for in-home supportive services. Objectives are to develop an in-depth client-service profile and provider inventory to examine the interface between providers and recipients; to design and test a system for the recruitment, training, and appropriate placement of in-home service workers; and to develop procedures to measure quality of care, including such elements as client functioning, outcome, and client/caregiver satisfaction.

VIRGINIA—The Commonwealth of Virginia Department of Medical Assistance Services was one of the first services in the nation to administer a preadmission screening program. It is believed to be one of the most effective programs in targeting nursing home applicants to the most appropriate and desirable care setting, with a reported accuracy rate of 60% in 1986. Administrators believe that this rate could have been higher if adequate services were available. The quality assurance model for community-based care has four components: preadmission screening, admission certification, monthly patient home visit by a provider RN, and a utilization review. All four components work together to provide structure, process, and outcome checkpoints and safeguards for the program.

WISCONSIN—Home care services are provided primarily at the county government level, with supervision and funding from the state government. The responsible state agency is the Department of Health and Social Services through its Bureau of Long-Term Support, Division of Health, and Division of Community Services. Quality assurance in Wisconsin's home care programs also is implemented primarily at the county level. The counties do not use Medicare's skilled home care quality assurance procedures in these programs; instead, they rely on a combination of case management, consumer grievance processes, an option for consumer supervision of providers, and county monitoring plans. Emphasis is placed on consumer satisfaction as an indicator of program success.

WYOMING—The Wyoming Community-Based In-Home Service Program operates under the auspices of the Wyoming Commission on Aging. Wyoming has sparse professional and community resources and a widely dispersed elderly population. Therefore, Wyoming has developed a Rural Social Case Management model that relies on paraprofessional case managers who operate under the direction of program directors usually based in multipurpose senior centers. Their role is to assess need, develop care plans, broker/purchase in-home care, and monitor and follow-up on clients and services.

With its safeguards of staff training, quality monitoring, and technical assistance, and its focus on client-specific services and outcomes, the Wyoming social model of case management is one that can be adopted in similar rural settings. It is not only a cost-and resource-effective service delivery alternative, preventing premature institutionalization of the frail elderly, but it also promotes the client's dignity and involvement in choosing and maintaining life-style preferences. In other words, it supports the client's perspective on quality of life and quality of care. Wyoming has recently applied for a Medicaid waiver to supplement Title III and state funding. The rural-social model is fully explained in chapter 8.

State Licensure of Board and Care Facilities

Statutes in all states, with the exception of Louisiana, regulate board and care facilities (BCF). Most states prescribe licensure, and a few also provide "certification" or "approval" of BCF or their programs by various payment agencies, such as developmentally disabled (DD) or mental-health-placement agencies. A major impetus behind state licensure was the 1976 enactment of the Keys Amendment to the Supplemental Security Income (SSI) program (42 U.S.C. 1382(e), P.L. 94-556, section 505d), which requires that states regulate admission policies, safety, sanitation, and resident civil rights in BCF where "a significant number" of SSI recipients do, or are likely to, reside.

Unfortunately, the only federal sanction to enforce the Keys Amendment is federal reduction of the amount of any state supplementary SSI payments for medical or remedial care to the individual clients—not the best incentive to increase regulatory oversight. However, as the U.S. General Accounting Office (1989) has noted, the Keys Amendment has been useful in that it has encouraged some states to regulate certain aspects of BCF operation. The American Bar Association has recently published *A Model Act Regulating Board and Care Homes: Guidelines for States* (Beyer, Bulkley, & Hopkins, 1984).

PUBLIC SECTOR REGULATION OF COMMUNITY-BASED HEALTH CARE: FEDERAL

Medicare Certification of Home Health Agencies

Medicare, the federally financed and administered program of health insurance for the elderly and totally disabled, provides only national public standards for community-based care. Its ten "Conditions of Participation" apply not only to the more acute types of home health care covered by Title 18, but also to home health care services under Medicaid. Briefly, the Conditions of Participation prescribe standards for agency organization and staffing, staff responsibilities, contracting with other persons and organizations, admission criteria, patient care planning, program evaluation, and record review.

Statutory amendments in the 1987 Omnibus Budget Reconciliation Act add additional requirements for patients' rights, ownership disclosure, aide training, in-service training, and patient assessment. In general, home health agency standards are more "process-oriented" than current nursing home standards because, to some extent, they examine care planning and actual care delivered to patients.

The Conditions of Participation are enforced through surveys by state inspectors required to interview a sample of patients as well as records and care-planning documents. Home care agencies that meet all the regulatory requirements, or whose deficiencies do not jeopardize patient health and safety, are certified eligible to participate in Medicare.

As of 1986, Medicare Peer Review Organizations (PROs) are required to investigate complaints regarding Medicare home care quality. PROs may recommend imposing monetary penalties or disqualifying agencies with serious quality deficiencies from further program participation.

Medicaid Regulation of Home/Community-Based Services

As noted above, federal Medicaid regulations require that home health agencies meet Medicare standards, but states are permitted to prescribe additional requirements for home health agency participation.

The Social Services Block Grant (SSBG)/Title XX Services

There are no federal quality standards for SSBG or even specific requirements that states have such standards. Because these programs often use case managers to assess and refer clients to packages of needed services, case managers play an informal quality assurance role (Riley, 1989).

Title III, Older Americans Act Services

Like SSBG, there are no federal requirements for state quality assurance; however, Riley's (1989) survey suggests that most state aging agencies consider case management to be an effective quality assurance mechanism. States vary in their systems for review of the quality of the case management service itself. As noted above in the public sector regulation section, there is considerable activity nationwide to initiate quality assurance systems. Much of this effort has been funded by the Administration on Aging.

Long-Term Care Ombudsman Program

Passed in 1981, the Rinaldo Amendment to the Older Americans Act requires that board and care homes be included in each state's Long-Term Care Ombudsman Program. The ombudsman is responsible for investigating complaints concerning nursing homes and other long-term care facilities regulated by the state. Ombudsmen serve as mediators rather than regulators. In fact, the law specifies that an ombudsman cannot be an agency that licenses or certifies long-term care facilities, including board and care homes (Dobkin, 1989).

Although originally created as nursing home investigators, since 1987, the ombudsmen have been responsible for board and care and other adult residential facilities as well. Alaska, Connecticut, Idaho, Maine, Pennsylvania, Wisconsin, and Wyoming have authorized ombudsmen to investigate complaints regarding home care. Minnesota passed similar legislation in 1989. Pilot projects in limited geographic areas have been funded by the Administration on Aging in Colorado and Virginia. The Administration on Aging is currently charged with reporting to Congress regarding ombudsman activities in board and care facilities.

PRIVATE SECTOR QUALITY
ASSURANCE AND ACCREDITATION

The Joint Commission on Accreditation of Healthcare Organizations (JCAHO). JCAHO has recently revised its standards for home care accreditation and extended its hospital-based home health agency accreditation program to freestanding agencies. These standards are both structural and process oriented in areas of home environment, nursing care, medications, enteral/ parenteral nutrition, infusion therapy, general nutrition, respiratory care, transfusion therapy, patient activity levels, physical, speech and occupational therapy, and psycho-social care. Standards include a few outcome measures such as client satisfaction. Surveyors use observation, interviews (including client interviews), and record reviews.

The National League for Nursing (NLN). NLN has operated an accreditation program for 20 years, primarily accrediting visiting nurses' associations and public health departments. Accreditation by either JCAHO or NLN is voluntary, and there has been little incentive to seek this credential; however, in early 1988 the Health Care Financing Administration proposed deeming home health agencies accredited by JCAHO or NLN as meeting Medicare standards. If this proposal is implemented, it would dramatically increase the interest in accreditation.

The National HomeCaring Council. The National HomeCaring Council was funded in 1988 to develop a national certification program for homemakers, home health aides, and other professionals. The standards that have recently been revised are primarily structural in nature (National HomeCaring Council, 1988). They include requirement of a quality assurance committee, written policies, personnel qualifications, training, supervision, and in-home patient assessment. Standards on clients' rights and the process of case management were added in 1988.

The National Hospice Organization (NHO). The National Hospice Association adopted standards for hospice care in 1978 as a means of focusing attention on the need for quality of care. The organization then lobbied Congress to provide funding for such care. In 1979, the Health Care Financing Administration authorized the funding of 26 demonstration programs; in 1982, the Tax Equity and Fiscal Responsibility Act was amended to provide hospice benefits to those that were Medicare eligible. However, not all hospices elected to pursue certification under the new entitlement program. In 1987, the NHO reported that 24 states and the District of Columbia had adopted formal licensure laws or regulations.

National Institute on Adult Day Care. In 1979, the National Institute on Adult Day Care (affiliated with the National Council on Aging) was formed in an attempt to standardize day care service and to check its unfettered growth. Only 26 states (including the District of Columbia) currently license or certify adult day care centers; 15 other states set standards for centers that receive state funding (Hughes, 1989). Only 12 states have no regulation whatsoever (Fisher & Donohoe, 1989).

SELECT Home Health Services of America. SELECT is a national association of independently owned and operated agencies that provides health care services at home, such as visiting nurses, physical therapists, and homemaker/home health aides. All SELECT affiliates volunteer to meet and maintain standards of quality care, and each affiliate must adhere to the code of ethics for home health care agencies. The purpose of SELECT is to foster and promote local home health agency credibility by establishing and maintaining uniform high standards of care and agency integrity. SELECT also helps the agency by

means of cost-effective professional marketing and community awareness services and creates an identity with a national network of home
health agencies that provide quality care.

The National Association of Residential Care Facilities (NARCF).
The National Association of Residential Care Facilities was incorporated in 1984 as a nonprofit association representing owners and oper-
ators of homes providing shelter, meals, and personal care to the elderly
and mentally and physically disabled. In 1987, NARCF began an
administrator and provider certification program, and provides information and training to improve the quality of care in residential facilities. Today there are over 40,000 licensed facilities in the country.

The American Association of Homes for the Aged (AAHA). AAHA is
a national association of over 3,000 not-for-profit community-based
nursing homes, continuing care retirement communities, homes for the
aging, and community service organizations. The AAHA offers a national certification program for retirement housing professionals that
includes an educational program in management and social-service
techniques.

The Continuing Care Accreditation Commission is a forum of AAHA
members from continuing care retirement communities working together to assess the adequacy of their operations; it offers information
to consumers and the general public concerning the integrity and quality
of these communities.

National Association For Senior Living Industries. This association
provides a network and certification for the for-profit living center.

Private Insurance. It is expected that private purchasers of long-term
care will demand levels of quality that far exceed current minimum
standards set by the government. These higher levels of quality will
require greater resources and greater flexibility. The best way for
providers to ensure that the dollars are there to pay for care is to work
with quality-minded insurers to develop long-term care insurance programs that integrate financing and delivery (Lyons, 1989b).

Miraculous Machines. A discussion of medically related home care
would not be complete without acknowledging the advent of high-tech
home care and some unresolved or unaddressed policy issues related to
this service. The rapid pace of innovation in portable life-sustaining
equipment and technology, combined with a growing need for cost
control, has created strong pressures for high-tech home care. Accordingly, the numbers of technology-dependent people (of all ages) who
are cared for at home has greatly increased.

In a report for the American Association of Retired Persons, Leader (1987) discussed home utilization of life-sustaining machines, such as dialysis, nutrition therapy (TDN), and ventilation, as well as antibiotic infusion therapy and chemotherapy. The report points to the quality concerns being addressed by those services provided by home health agencies even though they are not the primary providers of high-technology service. Ironically, it is the suppliers of pharmaceutical, nutrition supplements, and durable medical equipment that are responsible for home service. Yet this service is unregulated to date.

The exploration of quality assurance programs is a complex extensive project that could be the topic of another book. As community-based long-term health care programs expand to keep pace with demand, their quality assurance plans are vital components to success for both clients and providers.

The chapters in the first section of this book reveal the complexity of community-based long-term health care; specifically, how it is supervised, subsidized, and certified. For the reader's convenience, all of the associations and organizations mentioned above are alphabetically listed in the appendix, along with their respective addresses and phone numbers.

The second section examines 12 models of community-based long-term health care. Each model has innovatively combined and coordinated the fragmented and complex components of care and costs into a working program.

SECTION II

Innovative Models

4

The Respite Care Center
Evanston, Illinois

with JOAN H. MOSS and RUTH FRIEDMAN

The Kellogg Respite Care Program, based in the north suburban area of Chicago, matches volunteers with a caregiver/recipient couple, providing four hours of breakaway time each week for the caregiver. The Evanston Hospital Corporation, Visiting Nurse Association North, and the College of Nursing at the University of Illinois at Chicago have collaborated to offer professionally managed respite care at no charge to the families.

PHILOSOPHY OF THE
RESPITE CARE CENTER

Respite care is a range of support services focused on the caregiver that provides temporary relief from the responsibility of caring for a physically and/or emotionally dependent individual. The goal of respite care is to sustain the caregiver relationship and enable the elderly individual to remain in the home or community setting.

The program encompasses a comprehensive array of services, including in-home and institutional-based respite care, information and referral, case management, client advocacy, and community and professional education activities. Central to the nurse-managed Respite Care Program is the referral of family caregivers to existing community resources, and case management services to families enrolled in the respite program. Community-based respite services in the home are provided by both trained volunteers and paid home respite workers.

Another program goal is education of professional, business and community leaders about the needs of the frail elderly and their care-givers. Most long-term care for the elderly is provided by family members at great personal and financial sacrifice. An advocacy effort to influence state and local policymakers regarding the need for more comprehensive long-term care policies and respite care are scheduled to be undertaken.

HISTORICAL OVERVIEW OF RESPITE

With a growing proportion of elderly persons in the U.S. population, caregiving for disabled elderly people is becoming a more frequent personal and social concern. Because of the pivotal importance of families in helping to maintain disabled elderly persons at home, the interest in family caregivers for dependent elders has become a major research and social service focus.

Respite Care. Care given to a disabled older adult in order to provide the caregiver temporary periods of relief from his/her caregiving re sponsibility has been a widely recommended service available to sup port caregivers. Some providers view respite as a natural outcome of traditional long-term services, while others view it as a separate and distinct service. Respite differs from other long-term care programs because it serves both the older person in need of care and the caregiver

Although formal respite programs are a relatively new concept in the United States, such programs were available in Great Britain since at least the early 1960s, when a "floating-bed system" evolved. This service allowed the temporary admission of the older adult to a hospital while family caregivers rested. In addition to providing respite to caregivers, these admissions created an opportunity for health care professionals to reevaluate the health status of the dependent older adult. This program offered a planned respite admission for two nights every two weeks, and could be combined with a hospital-based day respite program. Many developed countries have created models to offer family caregivers both planned intermittent respite care in the home or a community setting and short-term, temporary, institutional respite to enable family caregivers to vacation. In such countries, respite services are financed through national health services funding.

In the United States, the debate for publicly financed geriatric respite care has been primarily focused on in-home respite service. The major exception has been the VA system, which in some areas of the country provides institutional respite. Some hospitals and nursing homes have started institutional respite programs on a private-pay basis.

HISTORY OF CENTER DEVELOPMENT

A survey of family caregivers in Evanston, Illinois, found that the first priority for such individuals was respite from their full-time roles. The study was initiated by nurse faculty at the University of Illinois College of Nursing who observed that families were confronted with a "major crisis" when caregivers became ill themselves. When caregivers are unable to help dependent relatives, it can spell trouble for community services as well as the family.

The Kellogg Respite Care Center was created in July 1988 by the W. K. Kellogg Foundation to develop a continuum of respite services for caregivers of the frail elderly. The respite care delivery model utilizes trained respite volunteers to provide regularly scheduled respite in the home, and a contractual relationship with long-term care facilities to provide overnight respite. The institutional respite service provides both respite care in a protective setting and an opportunity for comprehensive evaluation of the elderly person's functional and clinical status. Services are coordinated and supervised by nurses.

ARRAY OF RESPITE SERVICES

The Respite Care Program provides in-home volunteer assistance and short-term, temporary admissions to cooperating long-term care facilities.

Referral Service. Trained staff are available to help families identify their needs for both medical and social services and for the referral of individuals to existing community resources.

In-Home Assessments for Respite Services. Caregivers interested in respite care programs receive a free assessment visit at home by a professional nurse, who helps the family discuss its needs for care.

In-Home Respite Care. Trained volunteers are available to provide most caregivers 16 hours per month of short-term, intermittent "relief" time in the caregiver's home. This service is without charge and provides the caregiver a much-needed break.

Institutional Respite Care. The Respite Care Project, in cooperation with the Presbyterian Home (Evanston), Brandel Care Center (Northbrook), and Brentwood North (Riverwoods), provides overnight respite care for up to three-weeks at one time. Respite admissions are coordinated by a nurse consultant. Limited funds, based on family income, are available to assist families with the room and board costs associated with this service for up to 14 days per year.

Respite Care Newsletter. A letter designed for caregivers, volunteers and friends of respite is published quarterly. Information about grant activities, recognition of volunteers, and articles of support for caregivers are featured.

Community Education Program. Project staff are available to community organizations for presentations on such topics as aging and health, community-based services for the elderly, and respite.

Professional Education. Presentations concerning various aspects of the program have been made to health care professionals and students.

FAMILY INTAKE PROCESS

Referral. Most families are referred to the service by the network of visiting nurse associations and social service agencies. Marketing efforts such as direct mail or paid advertisement in local papers have been largely ineffective. Family caregivers are unfamiliar with the terms "respite" and "caregiver." Caregivers need more than a description of the service. They need professional support to consider the benefits for both themselves and the care recipient. Other successful referral sources include adult day care programs, senior centers, caregiver support groups, and hospital discharge planners.

Eligibility. Eligibility criteria for the Respite Center include residence in a defined geographic service area (primarily determined by the size and location of the volunteer coalition); age of the care recipient

(65+); presence of a family caregiver in the same residence as the older client; inability of the family to leave the elder person alone for extended periods (e.g., more than one hour); and the appropriateness of a trained volunteer to safely provide care.

Intake Procedure. After an initial phone screening for eligibility by a registered nurse, a home visit is scheduled. The intake assessment includes data on both the caregiver and the recipient. Demographics, medical history, medications, utilization of other formal and informal services, caregiving training, functional assessment of the care recipient, and the psychological and social impact of caregiving on caregivers are some of the general areas included in the intake assessment. The preferred type and frequency of respite is also discussed. Most families prefer a weekly home respite visit (4 hours), allowing caregivers an opportunity to socialize with friends, run errands, and/or seek health care services for themselves. The minimum number of scheduled respite visits is one visit per month in order to enhance the continuity between family and volunteer.

Volunteer/Family Match. Volunteers select their family assignments with the expectation that respite will facilitate an extended relationship (often 1 to 2 years) between the family and themselves. Factors considered in the matching process include volunteer availability; family's preference for day/time, educational, occupational, and cultural background; age preference; and volunteer comfort with functional needs and required assistance. A paid respite specialist is available to provide respite visits for up to 8 weeks in the event a trained volunteer is unavailable at the time respite is requested.

Case Management. The case management component of the respite program is the comprehensive assessment, development, and evaluation of an individualized family management plan to support families caring for a frail dependent elderly person in their home. The unique characteristics of the case management approach include:

- a focus on the family unit over time;
- assessment of health/nursing needs;
- social and psychological concerns; and
- actual provision of respite services in the home or institutional setting under supervision of the nurse case manager.

The history of chronic illness and frailty of the elder clients causes constant changes in health status. This often necessitates that case managers, as part of their intervention role, provide nursing care to both caregiver and care recipient.

Evaluation and Monitoring. Evaluation and monitoring of the respite intervention for both family and volunteer is provided by the same professional nurse who completed the intake assessment. The continuity of the nurse/family/volunteer relationship is a critical element to the project's success. The family sees the nurse's role as both supportive and supervisory to the volunteer's work, and as a knowledgeable resource for other health and social services as those needs arise.

Termination of Service. Most respite services are terminated because of care recipient death (45%), permanent institutional placement (25%), or when the recipient leaves in order to stay with his or her family. Volunteers may choose to continue seeing the caregiver for a month after the service has ended in order to offer support to the family. Approximately one-third of the families (35%) complete the project annually.

VOLUNTEER PROGRAM

Volunteers provide nearly all the respite care in this community-based program. There are currently 48 volunteers (three of whom are men), providing over 450 hours per month of direct respite service to families. The age range for volunteers is from 25 to 82 years, with a large number either in their twenties or above 60 years of age. Approximately 25% of respite volunteers are active older adults whose central motivation to volunteer is meaningful productive activity and social interaction.

VOLUNTEER ROLE

Volunteers in the program do not view themselves as baby-sitters but as individuals who provide a therapeutic service for the homebound older adult. Volunteers sometimes use prepackaged "visit kits" to help them structure a therapeutic activity for a visit. In addition to providing time away for the caregiver, volunteers provide social support to the caregiver by making time for active listening or sometimes helping out with an unexpected errand. Most of the volunteers form close relationships with the caregiver, especially when the caregiver has a limited network of support. This relationship may continue after the family is no longer in the program due to the death of the older adult. The in-home respite program strengthens and facilitates the family's informal network of care, with professionals acting in partnership with community members.

Volunteers are part of the case management model of the program. Because volunteers see the clients on a regular basis, they are often the first to notice changes in the caregiver or care recipient. Volunteers report these observations to professionals within the program or encourage the caregiver to contact the program so that appropriate help can be given. Early intervention can occur before a situation becomes a crisis or leads to more serious disability.

VOLUNTEER TRAINING

Volunteers participate in an initial 12 hours of training. The training includes sessions on the following:

1. orientation to the concept of respite, the mission and services of the Kellogg Respite Care Program, and the roles and limitations of volunteers within this program;
2. overview of aging including physiological, developmental, and social aspects;
3. skills of therapeutic communication;
4. family dynamics and community resources;
5. safety issues, including transfer techniques, assistive devices, and environmental factors in the home setting; and
6. diversional activities that provide stimulation for homebound older adults.

After the initial training in a group, all volunteers receive at least one training session in the home of the family with whom they are matched. Depending upon the skills of the volunteer and the needs of the older adult, additional training may be arranged.

Client Registry. In preparation for the respite visit, volunteers are given both a client registry sheet and a respite care plan for the family.

The client registry sheet has general and basic information that is essential in case of an emergency. If emergency medical help is required, this information can be given to the paramedics. It has proven

Kellogg Respite Care Project
Client Registry

Client Information

Caregiver Name_____ Registration Date_____

Relationship to Care Recipient_____

Length of Time as Caregiver_____

Other Persons Living in the Home_____

Home Address_____

City, State, Zip_____

Home Phone_____ Business Phone_____

Emergency Information

Doctor_____ Phone_____

Hospital_____ Phone_____

Emergency Contact: Name_____ Phone_____

                    Relationship to Client_____

Care Recipient Information

Name_____ Date of Birth_____

Type of Disability_____

Services Desired_____

Diet_____

Medication_____

Adaptive Equipment_____

Communication_____

Hobbies and Interests_____

Special Needs_____

In Case of Emergency:

Your Community Emergency Number is

_____

AND... You can always reach a respite staff nurse by calling **708/570-2000** and asking to page the "on-call" staff member on the long-range pager.

Figure 4.1. Kellogg Respite Care Project Client Registry. Used with permission.

Kellogg Respite Care Project
Volunteer Job Description

PRIMARY FUNCTION

The Respite Care Project Volunteer functions as a companion or trained visitor to families who provide care to frail dependent elderly persons. Volunteers do not provide skilled care but are expected to perform routine, custodial and diversionary tasks.

VOLUNTEER ACTIVITIES

- Provide a safe environment and basic physical care for an older adult while caregiver is out of the home.
- Provide support for family caregiver by active listening
- Engage in socialization and diversionary activities with the older adult during the respite visit.
- Share information about available community services with caregiver
- Communicate new or changing needs of the family to the Community Respite Director.

HOURS

- Schedule to be arranged
- On average a respite visit is 4-5 hours

QUALIFICATIONS

- Sincere interest in working with the frail elderly and their families
- Patience, good humor, flexibility, reliability
- Ability to maintain confidentiality
- Communication skills—both a good conversationalist and a good listener
- Successful completion of the volunteer training program

BENEFITS TO VOLUNTEERS

- Community service
- Career exploration
- Experience for future career in gerontology (may receive written references as needed)
- Personal satisfaction from helping others

Figure 4.2. Kellogg Respite Care Project Volunteer Job Description. Used with permission.

to be helpful in guiding volunteers through emergencies. In a medical emergency, volunteers may have trouble remembering their location by a specific address and the community emergency number. Volunteers bring the client registry sheet with them for each respite visit. A respite care plan is also available that describes individualized information as to what should be done during a respite visit.

Continuing Education. Continuing education programs are held on a regular basis to enhance personal development of the volunteer. One of the program goals is the development of credible and knowledgeable leadership in communities concerning the issues of maintaining older adults in the community and long-term care. In addition, these educational programs are organized to provide an opportunity for volunteers of different age groups to socialize with one another. The interaction between different age groups of volunteers may help to dispel a view of aging that focuses only on dependence or illness.

FINANCIAL COMPONENT
OF RESPITE CARE CENTER

The Respite Care Center has been established as a demonstration project funded by the W. K. Kellogg Foundation. The grant is supported by three agencies: the Evanston Hospital Corporation, the Visiting Nurse Association North, and the University of Illinois at Chicago, College of Nursing. Their collaborative support and expertise demonstrate the need for private and public sector commitment to address the long-term care needs of the elderly and their families.

Volunteers. The program utilizes both stipend (25%) and nonstipend volunteers (75%) to provide in-home respite. Our experience with elderly volunteers is that this volunteer pool may need a small stipend ($2.25/hr.) to offset the costs associated with their volunteer commitment (e.g., transportation). In return, the project gains reliable volunteers available to provide many hours of care. In fact, the stipend senior volunteer group (12 members) provides two-thirds of the total respite hours provided by the project. Staff support includes 1.5 FTE (full-time equivalent) registered nurses and 0.5 FTE secretary. Nurses administer the program, including the recruitment, training, and supervision of volunteers; family assessments; volunteer and family matching; and case management. Indirect support, such as office space and phone expenses, are donated by the supporting agencies. Long-term financing of the program will be built on a mix of private-pay (25%), agency support (50%), and foundation or community organizations support (25%).

Community Support. Community involvement is the lifeblood of the Respite Care Program. Both individuals and community groups offer expertise needed to support the continuum of respite services offered to family caregivers.

The Junior League of Evanston and Volunteer Bureau of Lake Forest and Lake Bluff have incorporated respite care into their missions of serving community needs through volunteerism. Junior League members have contributed to the Respite Care Center through the development of a community education program regarding respite care and as in-home respite volunteers.

The auxiliary of the Evanston and Glenbrook hospitals also supports creative programs that contribute to the welfare of the community and increase public understanding of the volunteer role. Auxiliary volunteers provide their support in various ways: transportation assistance for respite volunteers, welcome gifts for families of the institutional program, and financial support of a community educational documentary video titled *Taking Care*. The videotape was produced by the Kellogg Respite Care Project and is available free of charge to community groups wanting to learn more about the issues of families caring for an older adult and respite care.

The Garden Guild of Winnetka has also found a way to support family caregivers through the program. As an organization committed to making the community more attractive, the Garden Guild regularly donates plants and other horticultural projects to homebound families in the program.

It costs $900 per family per year to provide a respite volunteer (based on 50 weekly visits of 4 hours). This includes the administrative costs of recruitment, training, and supervision of volunteers; family assessments; transportation; volunteer stipends (for senior companions); and secretarial support.

EVALUATION OF RESPITE CARE CENTER

Evaluation of the respite care demonstration project will focus on community utilization of the respite services; analysis of the caregiving relationship and the impact of respite services on the caregiver and frail elderly; and the effect of the project on community long-term care planning and policy initiatives.

A comprehensive evaluation plan has been designed to gather information that will be used to consider the effectiveness and worth of the respite interventions. Specific caregiver outcomes under study include perceived burden, the impact of caregiving on physical and mental health, stress, quality of life, and desire to institutionalize. Demand for services and family utilization patterns are also being evaluated.

REPLICATION TIPS

- Initiation of respite services must begin with an assessment of community support (e.g., interest in developing the volunteer coalition) and caregiver need (including barriers to service utilization).
- Building a coalition of home care agencies and service-oriented community organizations has been an effective strategy to recruit volunteers and identify families with caregiving responsibilities.
- Newspaper advertising and direct mail have been ineffective; professional and social service agencies are important family referral sources.
- Families are hesitant to accept respite services; therefore, significant staff time is initially required to support acceptance of the service and trust of the volunteers.
- Professional nursing management of the service is essential because of the changing medical status and functional level of the frail elderly care recipient.
- The continuity of the volunteer/family relationship enhances volunteer retention and caregiver satisfaction with the service.
- Institutional respite is the least preferred type of respite, most often being used for vacations, out-of-town family events, or medical emergencies/hospitalizations.
- In-home respite is the respite intervention most preferred by families. It has a demonstrated positive impact on caregiver well-being, acceptance of other health/social services, and reduced desire to institutionalize the care recipient.

Ninety percent of the Respite Care Center services are utilized by eligible clients. This is significantly higher than the under 50% utilization rate reported in the respite literature. It is believed that case management is an important factor in the acceptance and utilization of service.

REFERENCES AND RESOURCES

For further information, contact:

Ms. Joan Moss, Project Director
The Respite Care Center
Burch Hall
2650 Ridge Avenue
Evanston, IL 60201
(708) 570-2633

5

The Five Hospital
Homebound Elderly Program
Chicago, Illinois

with WANDA J. RYAN

The Five Hospital Homebound Elderly Program is the only program in Chicago that provides long-term care for homebound, chronically ill elderly people, regardless of their ability to reimburse the program for its services. It is a community-based, not-for-profit agency that provides home health services as an alternative to hospitalization or nursing home placement.

Despite common perception, only about 5% of the elderly live in nursing homes at any given time. The vast majority live quietly—often forgotten and abandoned—in their own homes and apartments.

In their isolation, and often their poverty, they cannot afford to seek regular health care and, at times, do not know how to take care of themselves properly. They forget to take needed medicine at the proper intervals. Some require help in basic hygiene or in paying their bills. They clearly do not thrive when living alone without assistance.

PHILOSOPHY OF THE
FIVE HOSPITAL PROGRAM

A description of an actual case history best illustrates the philosophy of the Five Hospital program.

A female patient is referred to the Department of Social Work by a physician. He happened to be on call the previous night when she was brought in by police, who were called because she was found lying on the floor of her room with bruises. No one knows what exactly happened, but one suspects any number of things could have occurred in the shabby rooming house that once was a gracious townhouse on one of Chicago's lovely North Side streets. The patient never responded sufficiently to tell anyone anything about herself, but from others it was learned she had become a recluse after retiring from her job of caring for children. She was alone. Her family, all of whom lived out of town, had not been able to convince her to move closer to them. From her belongings, one could tell she'd lived very sparsely, and there were signs of mental deterioration. Religious poems, scribbled on sugar wrappers, filled her well-worn purse, as did Oklahoma oil rights.

This true case history is often repeated, with variations, in hospitals day after day around the country. One can become immune to such broken lives and rationalize that such individuals are no longer useful to society, or one can be sensitive to the pathos, rationalizing that it is a shame such situations exist but nothing can be done. Or one can attempt to bring about change. The Five Hospital Homebound Elderly Program is an attempt to bring about change and offer hope.

The mission of the Five Hospital Program is to:

- deliver comprehensive high-quality home health services on a cost-effective basis to the homebound elderly, enabling them to live independently in the community and to avoid unnecessary or premature hospitalization or nursing home placement;
- provide continuity of care to the homebound, utilizing a multidisciplinary team of health care professionals and volunteers in accordance with an individual plan of care for each patient;
- provide, within the program's capacity for charity care, home care services to individuals regardless of their ability to pay;
- allow corporate members to have continuing relationships with patients served by their hospitals; and
- provide leadership in home health care research, training, and education.

There are two components to the program's mission: short-term care, which allows patients to recover at home after hospitalization, and long-term care, which enables elderly clients to live out their lives in dignity at home. By taking advantage of community support systems, patients avoid chronic neglect, frequent hospitalization, and unnecessary or premature institutionalization.

HISTORY OF DEVELOPMENT

The Five Hospital Homebound Elderly Program was initiated in 1976 as a cooperative effort of five voluntary, independent, general hospitals located in the Lincoln Park-Lakeview area of Chicago. The social work directors of these North Side hospitals (Columbus-Cabrini Medical Center, Grant Hospital of Chicago, Saint Joseph Hospital, and Health Care Center) decided to do something about the plight of homebound elderly patients. They were disconcerted by the fact that the same elderly patients were making repeated visits to their emergency rooms. What these chronically ill elderly needed was ongoing preventive health care that would ensure that they received the necessary medical care and, therefore, might avoid repeat hospitalizations and unnecessary or premature institutionalization.

Clients who were accepted in the program were required to:

1. be 60 years of age or older;
2. reside in the geographic area served;
3. be homebound and medically underserved; and
4. be able to manage independently in the absence of 24-hour supervision from family or friends.

Client Assessment. All clients were assessed at intake by a nurse-social worker team that developed an individualized care plan with the client and the informal caregiver, if available. Clients who could not travel to obtain ambulatory care and whose physician did not make home visits were assigned to an attending physician from one of the five hospitals. The physician performed an initial physical examination and history, visited on a regular basis as necessary (once every 3 to 6 months, on the average, once the client was stabilized), and also followed that client in and out of the hospital as needed. Other care services included geriatric reassurance and volunteer services. A variety of other services, such as physical therapy, podiatry and laboratory tests, were also provided on either a contract or referral basis.

In contrast to Medicare/Medicaid reimbursement programs in 1976, no prior hospitalization was required for acceptance to the program, nor was there a limit on the number of service visits that could be provided. However, because the program operated on a fixed budget, its staff attempted to provide a minimum number of visits per client consistent with the client's needs.

Consortium Effort. The Five Hospital Homebound Elderly Program (FHHEP) was organized as a not-for-profit corporation by a consortium of five voluntary hospitals of Chicago's North Side. Rather than providing five separate home care programs within a two-mile radius, FHHEP's organizational structure allows the provision of long-term care to some 500 chronically impaired elderly in an efficient, economical manner. The program is community based in an apartment building that leases to the handicapped and elderly, with medical staff and business services provided by the five hospitals.

DESCRIPTION OF SERVICES

The founding president of the program was the late Leo J. Carlin. Sponsoring hospitals are Columbus-Cabrini Medical Center (two hospitals), Grant Hospital of Chicago, Saint Joseph Hospital, and Health Care Center. Policy is made by an 18-member board of directors that is made up of hospital representatives (50%) and community citizens (50%). The program's board of directors, an unpaid all-volunteer board, oversees the program and establishes the board policies under which it operates. Six members of the board are appointed by the sponsoring hospitals, while the other members are elected at large. A professional advisory committee has also been formed to review and approve the program's clinical policies and procedures. The committee provides medical advice and expertise needed to provide quality home health care.

Volunteers. An associate board of 50 community volunteers works to ensure funding, community relations, and patient visiting. Care is provided by a team that includes a physician, nurse, social worker, home health aide, and, often, a community volunteer.

Client Environment. Many program clients live in dreary, dangerous surroundings. Alcoholics and drug users inhabit the same buildings. Some of the buildings are dirty, ill-kept, and rapidly deteriorating. However, the older persons who live there seem to prefer such surroundings to the antiseptic, secure environment of an institution. They prefer to stay at home where they are comfortable and have a certain sense of freedom.

The Five Hospital Program makes long-term, and, where possible, lifetime, commitments to these people. The program's staff are still serving some of the original clients with whom they contracted when the project began.

ARRAY OF FIVE HOSPITAL PROGRAM SERVICES

Services available through the Five Hospital Program include:

Attending Physicians	Dentists
Skilled Nurses	Rheumatologists
Intravenous Therapies	Podiatrists
Social Workers	Ophthalmologists
Home Health Aides	Optometrists
Physical Therapists	Beauticians
Occupational Therapists	Community Health Nurses
Speech Therapists	MedCall Emergency Response
Nutritionists	Legal and Tax Assistants
Psychologists	Visiting Volunteers
Homemakers	Respite Care

Services are provided through a health and social services care team. Basic medical and social supportive comprehensive services are provided in the following manner:

Patient Identification and Referral. The program office serves as an intake center for persons seeking admission to the program. Initial inquiries are accepted from all sources.

Medical and Social Evaluation. Each patient receives a complete evaluation and assessment of need by the home care team of social worker and nurse prior to acceptance into the program. This assessment includes data regarding client functioning at the time of entry into the program. A care plan is then developed for the individual patient. This plan of care is subsequently reviewed and updated at periodic structured case conferences.

Home Medical Care. Patients requiring the services of a physician for evaluation and ongoing care are provided with such services in the home as part of the care plan. Services in the home by such specialists as podiatrists, ophthalmologists, or dentists are arranged as needed. Skilled nursing care, monitoring, and supervision are also provided where indicated.

Personal/Homemaker Services. Geriatric home health aides provide such paraprofessional nursing services as bathing, dressing changes, temperature taking, pulse monitoring, and certain rehabilitative services. The geriatric health aide also provides such services as light housekeeping and chores, shopping, meal preparation, and clothing maintenance.

Personal Consultation. In carrying out the prescribed care plan, the social worker provides the patient with counseling and consultation on social and/or emotional problems and arranges for, or refers for, supportive services not offered by the program.

Coordination of Services. The team attempts to assure that each patient will obtain the services necessary for continued care and maintenance at home. In addition to the direct services of the program, the team calls upon specialized health care services offered by each of the participating hospitals and other community resources, such as home-delivered meals, transportation, nutritionists, and protective services. Responsibility for coordination is carried by the nurse or social worker, depending upon the nature of the individual client problem.

Continuity of Care. The program has the full backup of facilities and services offered by the five participating hospitals. When hospitalization or special diagnostic and therapeutic services are required, the patient is referred to the appropriate participating hospital(s). In addition to managing the illness or disease that initially prompted the care, the home care staff spends a great deal of time monitoring how the patient is functioning at home, determining whether or not the home environment is conducive to the patient's thriving, and seeing whether the necessary supports are available for daily living.

Home care is recognized by the program to be a very personal matter. Assistance with such tedious tasks as hygiene and grooming, bathing, and attending to related needs requires a person who is sympathetic and is seen by patients as one who really cares about them. Besides all their hard work for the Five Hospital Program, many of the staff members volunteer on their own time to deliver Meals on Wheels on holidays and help other social service agencies in the community dealing with problems of the elderly.

Referrals. Referrals are made to the program by 50 hospitals, private physicians, families, social service agencies, and religious organizations. If the program's services are not appropriate for the prospective patient, the staff attempts to locate an alternative placement.

Profile of a Patient. A recent analysis of the program's patient data provides a profile of its typical long-term care client: female, age 83, living alone in a rented apartment, with $563 in monthly expenses. She has $523 in monthly income, 90% of it from Social Security, and $4,169 in financial reserves. She has chronic circulatory and arthritic conditions, and is seen regularly by a nurse and social worker. Over 94% of the long-term care clients receive no support from their families, and rely on the Five Hospital Program to maintain their independence.

Volunteer Component. Effective volunteers are an important part of what makes the Five Hospital Program so special. Twenty-five volunteers give of their time and talent to visit the program's long-term care patients. The volunteers' primary purpose is to eliminate some of the loneliness and isolation felt by patients who live alone.

Training Opportunity for Student Nurses. Nursing students from the Trinity Christian College in Palos Heights gain practical experience in community home health through the Five Hospital Program. Program nurses supervise students who spend 2 days per week for 5 weeks making home visits to some of the program's clients. The students teach patients about good health practices, assess and monitor chronic health problems, and provide selected direct care services.

Both students and patients benefit from this relationship. Students learn to be understanding, sensitive, and compassionate professional nurses by being exposed to the loneliness, depression, dependency, isolation, poverty, loss, and grief of their elderly patients. This experience helps prepare them to deal with the psychosocial concerns of their patients, as well as chronic medical problems. Patients benefit as they receive extra nurse care at no additional charge. The program benefits by greatly extending the amount of care, and students keep the nursing staff open to new ideas and trends in the health care industry.

Respite Care Component. The Five Hospital Program, along with five other area service providers (Council for Jewish Elderly, Japanese American Service Committee, Jewish Family and Community Service, Metropolitan Chicago Coalition on Aging, and Mount Sinai Hospital Medical Center), is participating in the Living At Home Project (LAHP). The focus of the LAHP is to provide respite to the caregivers of dependent elderly persons. This respite care can prevent premature placement of frail elderly persons in institutions by providing direct service to the older person while at the same time supporting the caregiver so the caregiving relationship can be effectively maintained.

The new respite program provides direct in-home services to the elderly and to the family, and provides education and training for responsible family members, providers of service, and volunteers. Caregivers need time to take care of themselves emotionally and physically. Through respite care and care training, LAHP is able to help sustain the caregiving role.

LAHP is sponsored by the Commonwealth Fund and the Retirement Research Foundation, and has expanded services to include the Volunteer Senior Companion Program; it has developed a multiagency caregiver support task force to provide training, information, and workshops.

Guardianship Service. Another task force (12 agencies, plus 2 state and 1 local Area Agency on Aging) has been created to develop a money management and guardianship service in Chicago. A Directory of Groups for Caregivers of Older Persons, plus a quarterly update of caregiver events, has been distributed. This multiagency consortium also allows the Five Hospital Program to locate the right services for a specific client and will soon have a computerized data base of all government programs for which a particular individual may be eligible.

Emergency Response System. For a minimal cost, Five Hospital Homebound Elderly Program patients can be provided a small, lightweight pendant or clip-on button. A touch of the MedCall button will quickly alert emergency service staff to assist the patient.

Programs for Well Elderly Persons. Two of the participating hospitals, Saint Joseph's and Grant, have initiated programs to help adults 65 years and older who are well to meet the challenges of aging. Both programs offer health education classes; lecture series; workshops; exercise and fitness classes; movies and video presentations; craft classes; support groups for stroke victims and diseases such as diabetes, Parkinson's, and Alzheimer's; special events, such as Olympic games and walk-a-thons; and even ice cream socials.

Membership also includes free travel planning service, preferred pricing on medicine and meals, physician referral, rehabilitative services, and help with Medicare claims.

THE FIVE HOSPITAL PROGRAM'S
FINANCIAL COMPONENT

Success at the Five Hospital Program is measured in the lives of elderly individuals who, with its help, maintain their dignity and independence at home. The program budget has grown from $116,200 in 1976 to $2,100,000 during the 1990 fiscal year. During 1989, the Five Hospital Program provided over 27,000 visits to homebound elderly patients. Eighty percent of the revenues of the program are based on a cost per unit of service, the unit of service being the home visit. The agency cost per visit Fiscal Year 1989 (excluding fund-raising cost and volunteer visits) was $69.36. The majority of the long-term care patients receive free services, costing the program $3,500 per year per patient. This compares with the average cost of $22,000 for a Medicaid patient in an Illinois nursing home. At present, there is no public reimbursement for long-term care and no likelihood of such in the immediate future.

Medicare and Medicaid. Medicare accounts for 59% of the program's yearly budget, with Medicaid picking up only 6% of the tab.

Charity. Charitable contributions from individuals, corporations, and foundations make up about 24% of the finances, while 10% comes from other nongovernmental sources.

The Five Hospital Foundation. The Five Hospital Foundation was created in 1986 to consolidate and give direction to the fund-raising efforts conducted on behalf of the Five Hospital Program. All charitable donations are channeled through the foundation, which conducts two special events each year: the humanitarian award dinner and another event decided from year to year. The award pays tribute to individuals whose leadership and community involvement reflect the program's commitment to helping others live with dignity and self-esteem.

Women's Board. In September 1986, Mrs. William G. Stratton founded the Five Hospital Program Women's Board, which has been responsible for an increasing amount of the charitable contributions received by the program through the annual spring gala and gifts from individuals, corporations, and foundations. In 1988, the Women's Board raised 30% of the program's charitable support. Obviously, funding is one of the keys to the continuation of the program. Every effort is made to obtain increased funding through:

- the building of voluntary support and contributions of individuals and foundations;
- third-party sources, such as Title XVIII and Title XIX, and private health insurance; and
- private-pay services.

Efforts will continue toward effecting changes in state and federal legislation so that expanded benefits may be realized. The program is following very closely the Pepper Commission proposal to provide home- and community-based long-term care services and protection against impoverishment of people.

EVALUATION OF THE
FIVE HOSPITAL PROGRAM

A 4-year follow-up evaluation of the Five Hospital Program assesses such outcomes as mortality, comprehensive functional status, and perceived unmet needs of its frail elderly. Major findings were significantly better in cognitive functioning and reduced unmet needs in the treatment group after 9 months. At 48 months, continued beneficial effects of treatment on cognitive status was observed. A trend toward more favorable outcomes, such as life satisfaction and perceived physical health, was also noted.

Despite savings in low-intensity of institutionalization, preliminary findings indicate the total costs of care were 25% higher in the home care treatment group. This add-on cost is accompanied by increased autonomy regarding locus of care and improved quality of life outcomes insofar as those in the treatment group who wished to remain at home were helped to do so (Hughes, Conrad, Manheim, & Edelman, 1988).

REPLICATIONS OF THE
FIVE HOSPITAL PROGRAM

In 1988, the Board of Directors committed the Five Hospital Program to expand its long-term care services to the Edgewater and Uptown neighborhoods. The board also reaffirmed the program's mission to deliver comprehensive high-quality home health services on a cost-effective basis to the homebound elderly regardless of their ability to pay.

REFERENCES AND RESOURCES

Hughes, S. L. (1982). Home Health Monitoring: Ensuring Quality in Home Care Services. *Hospitals 56* (21):19-47.

Hughes, S. L., Conrad, K. J., Manheim, L., & Edelman, P. L. (1988). Impact of long-term home care on mortality, functional status, and unmet needs. *Health Services Research 23* (2), 269-294.

Hughes, S. L., Manheim, L. M., Edelman, P. L., & Conrad, K. J. (1987). Impact of long-term home care on hospital and nursing home use and cost. *Health Services Research 22* (1), 74-80.

Kirkpatrick, Thomas B., Jr., President and Chief Executive Officer for the Five Hospital Program. See below for address and phone number.

For further information on the Five Hospital Homebound Elderly Program, contact:

Chief Executive Officer
Five Hospital Homebound Elderly Program
600 Diversey Parkway, Suite 200
Chicago, IL 60614
(312) 549-5822

6

The Block Nurse Program
St. Paul, Minnesota

with MARJORIE K. JAMIESON

A National Innovation Awards Winner, the Block Nurse Program has a neighborhood focus, drawing upon professional and volunteer residents to provide home health care for local elderly who might otherwise become nursing home residents. The value of the Minnesota program is reflected in awards from "Neighborhoods, U.S.A."; the Midwest Alliance in Nursing; Minnesota Governor Rudy Perpich; Harvard University and the Ford Foundation: "Innovations in State and Local Government"; and the Ramsey County Board of Commissioners.

DESCRIPTION OF THE BLOCK NURSE PROGRAM

The neighborhood focus of the Block Nurse Program means that all persons providing home health and long-term care live in the neighborhood the program serves. The county public health nurse service hires the nurses and home health aide/homemakers who live in the community, and therefore provides personnel service, quality control, and all administration. Even the members of the board of directors of each Block Nurse Program live in their respective neighborhoods.

PHILOSOPHY OF THE
BLOCK NURSE PROGRAM

The Block Nurse Program is based on the premise that keeping people at home and out of institutions enhances their quality of life, enriches neighborhoods, and reduces costs. The program endeavors to provide quality, cost-efficient, long-term home care at the local level with local health care providers. This decentralized model is a promising example of how community initiative can redesign service delivery for the frail elderly to provide more effective care at less cost.

The cornerstone of the program is the enhancement of the family's ability to meet the needs of its members. The program organizes and supports family resources, supplementing them with a mix of services from the neighborhood that includes: nursing, counseling, transportation, bathing, errands and chores, and physical therapy. These services are coordinated under the supervision of a public health nurse who holds the belief that the community is the public health nurse's client. The program, as established in its bylaws, has four purposes:

1. To establish a neighborhood-based service system using neighborhood professionals and volunteers to provide directly, or coordinate with appropriate agencies and resources, those health and social services needed by residents 65 and over;

2. To demonstrate a model of long-term care and health promotion that enhances the quality of life for St. Anthony Park residents, enabling them to remain in their own homes and avoid unnecessary or premature institutionalization;

3. To demonstrate a cost-effective model of long-term care; and

4. To promote the concept of neighborhood-based long-term care, and to assist in the replication of the Block Nurse Program in other neighborhoods.

HISTORY OF THE BLOCK NURSE
PROGRAM DEVELOPMENT

The community of St. Anthony Park in St. Paul, Minnesota, has about 7,000 residents, 12.5% of whom are 65 years of age or older, and an innovative program designed to provide nursing and other services to elderly neighbors at risk of being admitted to nursing homes. This community has demonstrated that a neighborhood can play an essential role in providing the coordination and access to services required by the elderly so that they may remain in their homes (Jamieson, 1990).

Insightful Nurse. A nurse conceived the idea that elderly people living in a neighborhood could receive health and social services from persons (professionals and volunteers) living in the neighborhood. Plans for the resourceful program began in 1981 when the need for an alternative health care and long-term care delivery system for elderly neighbors led a group of St. Anthony Park nurses and community council members, a social worker, and a state legislator to begin meeting to organize the Block Nurse Program. These concerned citizens recognized that many elderly are placed in hospitals and nursing homes unnecessarily when they could remain in their homes and receive satisfying, relatively inexpensive care from nurses, home health aides/homemakers, and volunteers living in the community. Efforts of family members could be supported and supplemented with an aggregation of neighborhood services that include nursing, personal care, peer support, transportation, homemaking, errands, and companionship.

Collective Attributes. The Block Nurse Program became a reality because the innovators had the right combination of personal characteristics, skills, background, and knowledge. These collective attributes include recognition of a need; adherence to a vision/mission; commitment of time and energy without expecting pecuniary gain; absence of self-interest; confidence to take many risks; fortitude and optimism to view the insurmountable as a challenge; wisdom to network and negotiate; the ability to give others credit; and maturity to facilitate interdependence by resolving conflict as it occurs.

Dreaming and brainstorming were done evenings and Saturdays; deliberations were unencumbered by the usual consideration of a job or a boss! In a collaborative, cooperative atmosphere, ideas were discussed and direction agreed upon, while rewards were intrinsic and set the tone for the entire project. The grueling detail work necessary to launch a new collaborative venture required the pooling of knowledge, experience, insight, and sensitivity from community-minded people who were unafraid to tackle an old problem in a new way.

Community Involvement. The innovators involved in this program were trusted community leaders who tended to be opinion makers, but who engaged the residents of the community in any change process.

Support from major actors who could facilitate change was sought. Careful thought was given to identifying and involving related entities in the community. It seemed wise not to alienate anyone. The neutralizing of turf began early, and the advice of many was asked often.

Organizers received much support and encouragement from the community through its district council. St. Paul has a Citizen Participation Process, a method that brings together people in each of the 17 districts to improve their neighborhoods and be part of the city government's decision-making process. Initiating projects is one of the responsibilities of these districts. Each district has an elected council, whose members discuss and act upon neighborhood issues, and a paid community organizer. In St. Anthony Park, the organizer is a member of the program's board of directors and serves as a liaison to the community at large.

Since program planners agreed that too much planning stifles, causing openness to change to evaporate, the program developed one step at a time. The planners constantly reminded themselves that they needed to resist being formed to fit into the present system. Small successes led to larger ones, and confidence grew, though there were many low periods and times of uncertainty. Zeal was tempered by tenacity—the tenacity it takes to learn how to write grant proposals, to "beg" for in-kind contributions, and to converse with legislators, funders, and bureaucrats threatened by change.

Shared Vision. The community planners shared a sense of caring and belonging. They had knowledge of the neighborhood, had personal relationships, and could act rapidly, accurately, and more acceptably because they dealt with local issues. They acted in the interest of the elderly by maximizing flexibility without imposing regulatory barriers. There is trust in a community when all share the same frame of reference and same values, and the setting of the neighborhood is safe, known and comfortable.

The Block Nurse Program is a joint venture between the local government entity and the Public Health Nursing Service. It is an innovative departure from the conventional service delivery system. No new agency has been established to operate the Block Nurse Program. The Public Health Nursing Service is accountable for services provided by the program, and the local government entity serves as fiscal agent for the program.

Administration. A board of directors for the Block Nurse Program plans and directs the program. Members are neighborhood residents and a representative of the Public Health Nursing Service. Many of the overhead and administrative functions associated with the nurses' employment are the responsibility of the county. However, the Block Nurse Program's program director interviews applicants, makes hiring recommendations, and, in collaboration with the County Public Health Nursing supervisor, monitors and evaluates staff. The program director convenes care conferences and generally manages daily operations of the program as a whole.

The director of volunteers reports to the program director and to the community human services committee, and recruits, trains, and monitors volunteers.

The primary block nurse is part of a team of public health nurses who serve the county and is responsible within that system; she reports to a supervisor at a decentralized public health nursing station. The supervisor reports to the central county public-health nursing service administration office.

ARRAY OF BLOCK NURSE SERVICES

Nursing services are usually available 24 hours a day, 7 days a week, depending upon available staff and total costs, and include any service necessary for maintaining an elderly person at home. Usually, block nurses and block companions (home health aides/homemakers) are available. Other times, backup staff from the Public Health Nursing Service are used. The primary block nurse has the responsibility and authority to arrange and coordinate service delivery in the client's home. Services provided and/or coordinated include case management, financial management, home maintenance, household management, housing options, medications, nursing services, personal care, psychosocial needs, rehabilitative services, respite care, and transportation.

Case Management. The case management component of the Block Nurse Program is designed to assist persons aged 65 and over and their families to promote and maintain optimum health and independence while living at home in the community.

Each client, together with family members, is responsible for making decisions about his or her own health. Every client is assessed by a primary block nurse, a neighborhood resident who is a certified public health nurse employed by the County Public Health Nursing Service. The nurse helps the client and family determine the services needed and develops a specific care plan. The nurse then either delivers care or assigns a block nurse (a registered nurse who also lives in the neighborhood) to teach and provide support to the family, and deliver, coordinate, and supervise care that the family cannot provide. All block nurses complete a course in gerontic nursing.

Assessment. The initial nurse assessment considers the client's health status by taking a health history (including hospitalizations and family history), a functional assessment, and an analysis of the client's family function, nutritional status, cognitive status, environment (safety), complexity of care, body systems assessment, and nursing needs.

Screening. The second stage entails screening for needs related to personal care, vulnerability, frailty, transportation, respite, socialization, homemaking, meal preparation, shopping, chores, pharmacy/grocery delivery, housing, home maintenance, and financial status.

The Care Plan. The Care Plan Development follows as health problems are identified. Clients are referred to a physician for diagnosis and treatment whenever necessary. Services needed in order to effectively manage health problems are specified, such as health education for life style change, nutrition, and exercise; health education for disease/disability control; medication management; and home health services. The second segment of the care plan specifies who will provide the services: the client and/or family, the block nurses, block companions (home health aides/homemakers), block volunteers, or other professionals from community organizations. When necessary, the plan coordinates physical therapy, occupational therapy, speech therapy, medical social service, mental health, and chemical dependency counseling.

Monitoring. An ongoing component of the case management model is the monitoring and supervision of the client, family, providers/block nurses, block companions, block volunteers, respite care, hospitalization, discharge planning, nursing home rehabilitation, and hospice care.

Block Volunteers. Neighborhood residents trained at a vocational-technical institute provide home health aide and homemaking services as block companions under the block nurse's supervision. Counseling and emotional support are available from block volunteers trained as peer counselors through a University of Minnesota program, and from church volunteers known as Befrienders trained by the Wilder Foundation.

Staff members and volunteers enjoy working in their own neighborhood and, therefore, remain in the program over time. Nurses, home health aide/homemakers, and trained volunteers live close by and are accessible to the client and family members. Staff members know the client and the neighborhood well and can, therefore, link resources and coordinate services efficiently.

The community councils represent the neighborhoods in city affairs and support the program. The council can form a key link in the network of neighborhood resources by acting as a fiscal agent, assisting in grant applications and fund-raising, or acting as an information source to the neighborhood.

Neighborhood youth (Scouts, 4-H, and church-related groups) contribute time for service projects, such as snow shoveling, painting, and yard maintenance. Neighborhood churches share their trained volunteer visitors with Block Nurse Program clients. Neighborhood citizens run the program—in other words, they find the nurses and recommend who to hire. They perform many volunteer activities, ranging from providing socialization to arranging grocery delivery, and providing transportation to the doctor, picnics, and concerts. Local businesses contribute financial and in-kind support to the Block Nurse Program.

Neighborhood residents who need help are identified in several ways: word of mouth from friends, contacts by churches and other community organizations, and referrals from hospitals, physicians, social service agencies, and neighbors. The program builds on neighborly interest in the well-being of local residents.

FINANCIAL COMPONENT OF THE BLOCK NURSE PROGRAM

The program is committed to using existing resources and agencies, and has not created anything new or a new level of management. For example, the program's relationship with the County Public Health Nursing Service, responsible for personnel and fiscal administration, enables the program to bill existing government and private payers for services eligible for reimbursement. The program uses existing agencies for services other than nursing, personal care, and homemaking.

In the pilot project, approximately 25% of the services were reimbursed by Medicare, Medicaid, or third-party insurance. However, Medicare and Medicaid restrictions are complex and numerous. Some home health services are reimbursed by Medicare, private insurance, or Federal Title XX. A state program exists to provide "alternative care grants" for home care for low-income persons who would otherwise require nursing home care.

Fees that are not reimbursed by one of the above sources are charged to the client on a sliding-scale basis that is determined by the individual's ability to pay. These fees account for an additional 25% of reimbursement. When clients cannot pay the full amount, charitable contributions from private funders are used to cover the difference. In the pilot community, this figure, administered by a local government entity, amounted to 50% in 1985. Of the 50%, county levy monies paid for 25% of the nonreimbursed nursing and home health services. The average monthly cost per client was less than $300 in 1985.

Client Contributions. A distinctive feature of the program is that the client pays for only the actual time spent in the home, without minimum fees or stipulations about the duration of service. This policy has led to lower cost of service to clients. Clients are billed according to their ability to pay, free service is provided if indicated, and all clients are accepted regardless of ability to pay or eligibility for reimbursement.

Gatekeeping. A common case management issue is gatekeeping, the ability of programs to assess real need versus unnecessary dependence. Block nurses are in a position to be effective gatekeepers because the program is focused on knowing the community and residents' needs. It seems much easier to address this issue from an informed vantage point established through community networks than through programs that are less in touch with the needs and circumstances of area residents.

Service Delivery. The primary block nurse case-managing function allows the nurse to authorize delivery of any service regardless of entitlement or criteria from the government or insurance companies. Flexibility has enabled:

- a fraction of an hour to be used for nursing visits, if this meets client needs (no minimum of time per visit); more than two hours of daily nursing care despite regulations specifying a two-hour maximum; delivery of services for more than three weeks when appropriate;
- expansion of home health aide and homemaker functions into one job description thereby allowing greater efficiency in utilization of these personnel categories;
- the addition of trained volunteers for meeting client-specific needs, such as socialization, support, and transport;
- payment for services usually not covered by Medicare and Medicaid;

- expansion of coverage for case finding services performed by professional neighborhood nurses;
- consideration of an individual's functional abilities, impairments, resources, and environment, and the provision of the right mix of services—not too much and not too little;
- needed services to be organized into a client-specific plan of care that can substitute for institutionalization.

Family Involvement. The Block Nurse Program tends to increase family involvement in the care of elderly relatives. In many ways, the program is set up to enable family members to stay involved with an elder's well-being and to become even more involved because they are not as burdened by the full responsibility for the elderly person's care.

Client Profile. The average client across all Block Nurse Programs is an 83-year-old female who lives alone and has no support system. Upon admission to the program, a nursing assessment is done to determine the client's ability to perform eight activities of daily living (ADLs). Preliminary data on 129 clients indicates that 45% need no help with ADLs (but usually require chronic disease management); 39.5% need help with 1, 2, or 3 ADLs (some require disease management); 8.5% need help with 4,5, or 6 ADLs (some require disease management); and 7% need help with 7 or 8 ADLs (some require disease management).

Specific ADL needs of the initial 108 clients in one community show that clients need help as follows: 47% with bathing, 20% with dressing, 19% with grooming and toileting, 13% with walking, 11% with transferring, 10% with eating, and 7% with moving in bed.

Average overall cost for block nurse services in this community for 1989 was $106 per month per client. Thirteen block volunteers have gone through various levels of training to do friendly visits and socialization and other activities. Thousands of hours have been contributed by the community in planning and implementing the model including monthly meetings of the community board of directors. A similar commitment of volunteer hours occurs at all sites.

In the three block nurse programs in St. Paul in 1989, the following reimbursement sources paid for the costs of direct services to clients in 1989: Veterans Administration, 2.1%; Medicare, 4.6%; Alternative Care Grant (ACG), 6.2%; county discount, 6.2%; client fees, 25.8%, and grants, 43.8%.

TRENDS

During the 7 years of the pilot and 2 years of replication in other sites, the following trends are surfacing, especially in the pilot site.

Bottom-Up Participation. Over 80% of the referrals come by word of mouth from the neighborhood. A "bottom-up" neighborhood participation endeavor seems more successful and better sustained than a "top-down" superimposed system. The community adapts the program to fit its needs without bureaucratic constraints. The community has become sensitized to the needs of the elderly and asks for group projects, such as church youth clubs, or as individuals concerned about a neighbor. The neighborhood furnishes its own informal quality control by contacting direct caregivers or the program director, all of whom are neighbors.

Client/Family. Families and family surrogates (usually neighbors) have become more involved with the elderly. Staff members report that the family's ability to meet the needs of clients is enhanced. Approximately 15% of the clients have elected to be discharged from nursing homes to block nurse care. People plan differently for their retirement when they know home services will be available. Of those clients who had died, some have chosen to die at home utilizing block nurse care.

Cost Effectiveness. Health education, prevention, and early intervention have prevented hospitalization for about 25% of the clients. Less time is spent managing care since all staff know the client and client support system. By combining home health aide and homemaker functions into one job description, greater efficiency is demonstrated. Staff are available during inclement weather or odd hours. Nurses often ski to client homes during snowstorms. Although a chart may be formally "closed," staff and volunteers often continue informal client contact; therefore, prevention is addressed. Also, the nurse can build upon the interventions and support that have previously worked with other clients.

EVALUATION OF BLOCK NURSE
PROGRAM PILOT

A 1985 evaluation of the St. Anthony Park pilot covering the period between October 1982 and June 1984 focused on three major areas:

experiences of clients in the program, opinions and perceptions of the St. Anthony Park Community and the professional health care community, and cost comparisons between home care programs and between block nurse services and nursing home care. Findings for each of these areas are described below:

Experience of Clients. Twelve clients, averaging 81 years of age, were interviewed. A diversity of needs was revealed, ranging from care for postoperative recuperation to daily, long-term skilled nursing care. The block nurse staff averaged 14.6 clients per month, and clients noted that receiving care from a nurse who is a neighbor made them more comfortable. Eighty-five percent of the Block Nurse Program clients would be forced to enter nursing homes if the program were not available. This fact was confirmed by the professional judgment of the primary block nurse, reviews of case records and documents, and reports of client family members. All indicators show that the Block Nurse Program tends to increase and enhance family involvement in the care of elderly relatives.

Community Perceptions. Community members expressed a sense of ownership of the program and were highly supportive of its efforts. This support was demonstrated through extensive volunteer commitment, which included board membership and direct service to clients. Nine dimensions were found to explain the qualitative distinctions between other home health care programs and the block nurse programs:

- client-centered programming
- coordination and integration of services
- community-based staffing
- prevention/recovery focus
- early intervention
- management of chronic illness/disability
- delayed or reduced institutionalization
- case-mix openness
- fee flexibility

There exists both a formal and informal community-wide outreach and communication system for dissemination of information. Communication through key community organizations and media is thoughtfully coordinated. The informal system is illustrated by the fact that over 80% of referrals into the Block Nurse Program are by word of mouth.

It was found that agencies and organizations typically have full agendas of their own and cannot supply the energy and time to create something new, though networking and personal relationships in the wider community have been capitalized upon and every contact and every organization has been looked upon as a potential advocate.

Cost Comparison. When compared to the fees of 14 St. Paul, Minneapolis, home care agencies, block nurse fees fell below the lowest found for registered nurse visits (when minimum hours were considered) and below the lowest found since the rate reduction for block companions. The total cost of living with Block Nurse Program care is at least 24% less than the minimum cost of a nursing home without nursing services. However, staff wages were equal to community standards. Primary and block nurses and home health aides and homemakers are paid according to County Public Health Nursing Service wage scale.

The average monthly cost per block nurse client was calculated to be $214 in 1985. The average monthly cost for skilled nursing care in a St. Paul, Minneapolis, nursing home was $2,100, while block nurse clients could be maintained at home with nursing services for less than $1,000 a month ($214 for block nurse services and an estimated $700 for mortgage/rent, food, utilities, and other living expenses).

After 7 years of providing services to elderly clients, the Block Nurse Program has found that services can be made available based upon the elderly's needs rather than eligibility for reimbursement. What is required is alternative funding, professional and volunteer community members, an informal network of family, friends, neighbors, church and civic groups, and service clubs, such as Boy Scouts and Rotary clubs.

REPLICATION OF THE
BLOCK NURSE PROGRAM

The Block Nurse Program has been granted more than $1.7 million by the W. K. Kellogg Foundation and the U.S. Department of Health and Human Services, Division of Nursing, to enable replication of the program in three diverse communities, two in St. Paul and one in Atwater, Minnesota, a town of 1,100 with surrounding farming areas. Replication will occur during 1988 through 1990 for a total of 1,000 clients. Approximately 65% of the funds are being used for nonreimbursable services and 35% for administration and evaluation.

It is hoped that the project will provide data to influence the formation of new public reimbursement policies and needed private insurance products.

For communities with an incentive to meet client needs in the home rather than in an institution, where quality and cost of services are important considerations, the Block Nurse Program offers an attractive alternative to more traditional public and private home care services.

In addition to financial benefits, the program has implications for improving the quality and responsiveness of public services, enhancing the self-sufficiency of families and neighborhoods, and heightening the intimacy with which care is given. The program suggests that neighborhoods could play a substantially larger role than they currently do in shaping and carrying out public services; that established public agencies and providers of innovative alternative services make better allies than adversaries; and that traditional definitions of public services need examination. Perhaps many public services could be "deprofessionalized," allowing for greater self-help and use of volunteers, and calling on specialists to perform only those tasks for which special training is required.

In addition to being a model of caring for the elderly at home, the Block Nurse Program could be adapted to meet other neighborhood needs: nursing and support services for new mothers or sick children, child care, education, and job counseling. Where skilled and caring people live together in communities and have neighbors who need help, many opportunities exist for responsive services based on the Block Nurse Program model.

Future Plans. The Block Nurse Program is concerned about older people who live elsewhere. The board of directors of the Block Nurse Program, Inc., seeks to influence public policy and insurance in long-term care using the Block Nurse Program as a model. Reimbursement incentives currently lie with hospital and nursing home care. Evidence that many neighborhoods can provide health and social services in the home at low cost and with an emphasis on education and prevention can be an important contribution toward change. Therefore replication and evaluation of the Block Nurse is in process.

As more and more people grow old and live many years beyond retirement, the quality and dignity of their lives will be an issue for every family. Good institutional care will remain an important need, but care in the home and within the neighborhood should be developed wherever possible.

Block Nurse Program planners agree that specific goals should be considered in order to:

- meet the elderly's needs to make staying home an alternative to institutionalization;
- include any person age 65 or older living in the district;
- use existing services, agencies, and resources;
- develop community commitment to the program;
- hire nurses, home health aides, and homemakers who live in the community, and pay them by community standards;
- enlist volunteers to work with professional caregivers;
- enhance the ability of the family care for its elderly;
- design a system in which as few people as possible deliver services in a home;
- bill existing government and private payers for services eligible for reimbursement;
- charge for only the actual time spent in the home without minimum charges;
- provide health education and prevention to clients; and
- collect facts and figures needed to improve the way care is delivered and paid.

Two basic tenets were developed: First, all clients, nurses, home health aides, homemakers, and volunteers live in the community. Second, no new agency was created; all appropriate existing resources and providers are used.

PRINCIPAL BENEFITS OF THE
BLOCK NURSE PROGRAM

Better Service. Care in the home is usually more satisfying and conducive to recovery than long-term care in an institution. However, without the Block Nurse Program, many elderly residents with temporary health problems or a general decline in health would have fewer alternatives to a nursing home.

Harnessing and Supplementing Resources. The Block Nurse Program makes care in the home possible in two ways. One is by harnessing and supplementing the resources of families to meet their own needs. The other is by identifying and responding to needs for help sooner than the traditional medical service system does, making it easier to remedy some conditions and to prevent others from occurring.

The Block Nurse Program draws on neighborhood resources not available to traditional health care providers, building on a spirit of community self-help to extend the family resources. The program draws on established training programs and institutions for a coordinated mix of volunteer, professional, and paraprofessional services. A comparable scope of service is not available from conventional health care sources. Those services that are available usually require a host of narrowly trained personnel to come into the home to perform particular tasks. The Block Nurse Program avoids such disruption and fragmentation by combining job descriptions so that only a few people are needed to perform a wide variety of tasks in one home, and by putting coordination and supervision of all personnel and support services under one individual, the primary block nurse.

Lower Costs. Three factors contribute to a lower overall cost of care. For people who can be helped to remain independent, care at home is less expensive than care in an institution. As calculated by an external 1985 evaluation, the cost of remaining at home with Block Nurse Program care is at least 24% less than living in a nursing home (mortgage/rent, utilities, food, and Block Nurse Program services are figured into the home cost).

In addition, the Block Nurse Program has developed methods to make in-home care less costly than is typically possible through the services of professional home care agencies. These methods include the use of local resources, savings on mileage and travel time cost, enhancement of the family's ability to meet its own needs, and the use of paraprofessionals and volunteers, all under the supervision of professional nurses. Only needed services in the amount necessary are provided. Finally, early diagnosis and treatment of health problems and prevention of more serious problems contribute to reduced long-term health care costs.

The fees for professional services under the Block Nurse Program are equal to or lower than fees for comparable services provided by conventional public and private agencies. For example, from 1986 until June 1989, a nursing visit cost $32. Some private nursing services offer a lower hourly rate, but they typically require a 4-hour minimum charge per visit, making the cost per case higher than that of the Block Nurse Program.

The nursing visit fee was increased to $50 on June 1, 1989, after a cost analysis by the County Public Health Nursing Service indicated that the true costs of the program were not being recovered by the county.

Negotiation between the Block Nurse Program and the nursing service included defining administrative and overhead costs incurred by the county as a result of its collaboration with the Block Nurse Program. Such costs not related to the Block Nurse Program were not figured into the new fee. Almost 91% of the projected 1990 county expense for the Block Nurse Program is for salaries, wages, and fringe benefits of program staff, as well as for a portion of the salaries of county supervisory and administrative staff involved with the program.

Nonreimbursable Services. In at least one respect, the Block Nurse Program incurs costs that the conventional delivery system does not. It provides nonreimbursable services (such as personal care) and services to individuals who do not qualify for reimbursement under current government programs or private insurance policies. Some of these costs are recovered through fees and others through charitable contributions. A case can be made that many of these services prevent a client's health or financial resources from dwindling to a point where the individual becomes the responsibility of the public and therefore the services represent a savings to the community at large.

Unlike the conventional medical delivery system, incentives under the Block Nurse Program favor maximum self-reliance and minimum use of costly professional services; early intervention and treatment of disabling illness; prevention and recovery rather than long-term treatment; and coordination and integration of services rather than fragmentation and specialization. To the extent that fees and charitable contributions cover the costs of services to nonqualifying individuals who need help, the program avoids incentives to institutionalize clients or to overdiagnose needs in order to obtain public or third-party reimbursements.

The replication project is currently demonstrating methods to improve access to nursing services in noninstitutional settings through nursing practice arrangement in communities. The ultimate goals of the Block Nurse Program are to design an appropriate service delivery model for the needs of the elderly and to create a new and more inclusive system for paying for health and long-term care.

REPLICATION EVALUATION

As replication progresses, it is imperative to obtain a valid data base documenting home-delivered long-term care use and cost, and to fill some of the information gaps of the insurance industry and pubic policymakers.

Elderly consumers have indicated a strong preference for home health benefits over nursing home benefits when considering long-term care insurance. However, insurance companies have been hesitant to liberalize benefits for home care for long-term chronic conditions because they lacked reliable utilization and cost data.

Public policymakers are concerned about the "woodwork effect"— that a great demand for LTC services will occur if more services are made available. A secondary concern is whether families will abandon their relatives if programs and services are added.

A recent evaluation of the three replication sites produced a wealth of sociodemographic data, a referral pattern, a client profile, and family involvement and service use and costs. The several data collection forms employed are briefly discussed below:

Sociodemographic Data. Data was compiled regarding where and how clients live, and their age, marital status, income, and family.

Assessment Data. Financial assessment determined whether clients were Medicaid eligible, while functional assessment addressed questions about how frail and dependent the clients were, their functional limitations, and case mix determination. The case mix system was established in Minnesota in 1985 as a reimbursement system for residents in nursing and boarding care homes certified to participate in Medicaid. The system has 11 payment classifications, A through K, based on care needs. With Block Nurse Program clients rated on the same scale as nursing home residents, cost comparisons can be made between home and institutional care.

Nursing Care Plan/Evaluation. This section used the problem classification system developed by the Omaha Visiting Nurse Association. It is a 44-problem system, divided into 4 domains of environmental, psychosocial, physiological, and health-related behaviors. The system was chosen because it was developed specifically for community nursing and is easily computerized. In the Omaha System, nursing interventions are categorized as teaching, guidance and counseling, treatments and procedures, case management, and surveillance.

Managed Care. Category III, Case Management, revealed time and cost of managed care of the frail elderly living in the community. Admission vital signs and pulse assessments were recorded; cognition was considered one of four problems that indicated a vulnerable adult. Next to each problem is an area for the care plan. This format allows information regarding the nursing process to flow from assessment, to plan, to intervention to evaluation on the same page. The flow sheet provides information on the length of nursing visits, the amount of indirect time associated with each visit, and the nursing category involved. This information is needed to tie costs to services.

Service Tracking Form. The Service Tracking Form is a record of services that are being provided to clients in their homes, and the providers, both formal and informal. Advisors from insurance companies want to know more about how much care is required to keep an elderly person with chronic health problems at home, who provides the care, and whether it is paid or unpaid work. The form lists 13 areas of service, and a provider code is entered for service tracking.

The Block Companion Weekly Report. The weekly report is a record of both hours worked by the home health aide/homemaker and services provided. Like the flow sheet for nursing, it allows a look at utilization and cost data for all clients, or any desired subgroup.

Data Collection. Block nurses collected data on 349 clients from the three replication sites (A, B, and C) and the pilot community. Community A is a town of 1,100 located 85 miles west of Minneapolis, with surrounding farming area. It has the lowest median family income and the lowest percent of population below the poverty level. Community B was the first community in Minnesota to replicate the model, starting services in 1987. It is the most affluent of the neighborhoods and has the highest percent of population age 65 and older. Community C, similar in population to Community B, has the highest percent of population below the poverty level. Its percent of population age 65 and older, 13%, is the same as Community D, the pilot community. According to the federal 1980 census, the national figure for population 65 years and older is 11%.

Sociodemographic Profile. The evaluation profiled the clients as being 65 to 101 years of age; the mean age at time of admission was 81 and the median age 82. Thirty-five percent of the clients were 85 or older. In Minnesota in 1980, 11% of all elderly people were over the age of 85, while the national figure was 8.9%. Thus the Block Nurse

Program is serving a significantly older population than the general elderly Minnesota population.

Block Nurse clients are less likely to have a spouse, and therefore a potential caregiver, than the larger elderly Minnesota population. Thirty-two percent of the clients were married; while almost half of the elderly in Minnesota in 1980 were married. Fifty-nine percent of the BNP clients live alone, compared to 29% of elderly Minnesotans living alone in 1980.

Fifty-one percent of Minnesotans own their homes. Many may eventually become eligible for Medicaid but will be reluctant to apply, fearing that their home ownership will be threatened. Will some of these elderly then go without monitoring or preventive care, perhaps precipitating a crisis requiring hospitalization or nursing home admission?

The sociodemographic profile also indicated that 99% of the clients are white; 53% have not graduated from high school; and 16% are college graduates. The major referral source is relatives and friends, indicating a trust in the neighborhood-based program.

The most common nursing diagnoses are impairments in neuro/musculoskeletal function, circulation, and pain, while 21% have a deficit in cognition. Perhaps the most striking piece of information is that 33% of the clients are vulnerable adults because of assessed deficits in caretaking, neglect or abuse, or cognitive impairment. This means there is much nursing time spent in communication with social services, family members, physicians, and others to assure that these clients live safely in their own homes.

Block Nurse Program clientele is one that requires assistance because of functional limitations. Forty-four percent of the clients are dependent in one or more activities of daily living (ADL). Bathing is the most common dependency, with 38% needing some assistance. Dressing and grooming are the next most common dependencies. Seventy-eight percent of the clients have a case mix score of "A", meaning that they have between zero and three ADL dependencies, no special nursing needs, and no behavior problems. In contrast, in Minnesota in 1989, 30% of nursing home residents were classified as As. Many of them could be living in the community with minimal assistance and at much less expense.

Family Involvement. The great majority of Block Nurse Program clients have involved families, and indication that the program is enhancing family care rather than replacing the assistance provided by family members. Thirty-three percent of the clients received social services of some kind, 24% received home-delivered meals, and 15% used transportation services.

Financial Sources. For 1989, the financial sources for direct and indirect client services average for A, B, and C communities break down as follows: client pay, 15%; community funds, 52%; county contribution, 8%; Medicare, 10%; Medicaid, 5%; Alternative Care Grant (ACG), 8%; and Veterans Administration, 8%. The average cost per client per month for Community A was $453; Community B, $235; Community C, $192; and Community D, $236. Community A, the rural site, had the highest percentage of Medicare (25%), probably due to the lack of competition for those clients. Community B, the most affluent of the three replication sites, had the highest percentage of client contributions (31%), which indicates that elderly people are willing to pay for a service they need and value. Community C has the lowest average monthly income ($579) and the greatest percent of population below the poverty level. Community funds made the highest contribution to care (79%) for Community C, with surprisingly low contributions from Medicare, Medicaid, and ACG.

Cost of Care. The average service cost per client per month ranges from $192 to $453. The average cost of a nursing home in the St. Paul, Minneapolis, metropolitan area is $2,200 per month. Adding an estimate of $700 living expenses to the service cost figures, the cost of living at home with Block Nurse care ranges from $892 to $1,153, less than half the cost of nursing home for most clients.

The Block Nurse Program has recently given the data described herein to the Minnesota Board on Aging and the governor of Minnesota. The next step is to share the data with policymakers, legislators, the insurance industry, senior citizens groups, health professionals, and others concerned about long-term care. This data will be combined with that of the Living at Home Project in St. Paul, a national demonstration funded by the Commonwealth Fund, in order to inform local, state, and national policymakers about neighborhood-based programs and the clients served, and to start building coalitions to support the concept.

REFERENCES AND RESOURCES

Campbell, J. L., & Patton, M. Q. (1985). External evaluation report of the St. Anthony Park Block Nurse Program. Unpublished report.

Community residents provide home care for elderly. (1984). *Hospitals, 58,* 54.

Jamieson, M. K. (1989). Nursing our neighbors. *American Journal of Nursing, 89* (10), 1290-1291.

Jamieson, M. K. (1990). Block nursing: Practicing autonomous professional nursing in the community. *Nursing & Health Care, 11* (5), 250-253.

Jamieson, M. K., & Campbell, J. (1987). The St. Anthony Park Block Nurse Program. *American Journal of Public Health, 77* (9), 1227-1228.

Jamieson, M. K., Campbell, J., & Clarke, S. (1989). The Block Nurse Program. *The Gerontologist, 29* (1), 124-127.

Jamieson, M. K., & Martinson, I. M. (1983). Block nursing: Neighbors caring for neighbors. *Nursing Outlook, 31*, 270-273.

Martinson, I. M., Jamieson M. K., O'Grady, B., & Sime, M. (1985). The Block Nurse Program. *Journal of Community Health Nursing, 2*, 21-29.

Selby, T. (1983). Block Nurse Program provides home care for older residents. *The American Nurse, 15*, 1-20.

For further information on the Block Nurse Program contact:

Executive Director
The Block Nurse Program, Inc.
Suite 125, Ivy League Place
475 N. Cleveland
St. Paul, MN 55108
(612) 649-0315

7

Rural Elderly
Enhancement Program
Montgomery, Alabama

with SHARON FARLEY

The Rural Elderly Enhancement Program (REEP) sponsored by the School of Nursing at Auburn University at Montgomery, Alabama, is a community-based program in Wilcox and Lowndes counties whose purpose is to develop support systems to help the elderly maintain their health and remain in their own homes and communities.

PHILOSOPHY OF THE PROGRAM

Many of the elderly in rural Alabama are poor, isolated, and have limited access to health services. REEP is a nurse-managed project that seeks to implement a model of community involvement, organization, and infrastructure development to improve the health and quality of life of some 1,000 rural elderly, who are primarily black and poor. The program works with local government units, agencies, volunteers, and schools to:

1. provide accessible and potable water and improved housing and transportation;
2. stimulate rural integrated development involving community coalitions, volunteer training, and public education; and

112

3. conduct assessments of the elderly and respond to their needs with linkage to services, training, respite care, and appropriate volunteer coalitions.

Some of the achievements of this project are:

- enhancement of independent living for the elderly;
- collaboration among community agencies;
- personal empowerment of elderly and county residents;
- training and job placement for low-income residents; and
- infrastructure improvement.

HISTORY OF DEVELOPMENT

The project was developed to assess and analyze needs of the elderly, develop community-based coalitions based on commonalities of needs, and link the elderly with appropriate coalitions and/or resources designed to provide support systems to keep the elderly in their homes and communities. While isolated support services were available, other services and mechanisms were needed to link the elderly with those resources.

Black Belt Area. The two targeted Alabama counties (Wilcox and Lowndes) are part of the 19-county Black Belt area, which got its name from the rich black soil found there. The predominantly rural area is located in south central Alabama and stretches across the state from Mississippi to Georgia. A majority of Alabama's black population lives in this 19-county region. (In Alabama, the percentage of black population is 25.6, while in target counties the percentage is 78 percent).

Continuing high unemployment, low-educational levels, and a high degree of dependency on public assistance programs have brought the target counties to be among the poorest in Alabama and the nation. The average per capita income in the target area is less than $7,300 compared to a national figure of $12,772. The counties report that about 60% of their population is at or greater than 100 percent of poverty level. Elderly blacks are more likely to be poor than whites, owing particularly to a faster decline in the occurrence of poverty among whites than blacks.

Medically Underserved. The U.S. Department of Health and Human Services has designated the Black Belt area as medically underserved and a health-manpower-shortage area. One of the targeted counties has no hospital or long-term care facilities and 1.5 physicians per 10,000 population. The other county has a 32-bed hospital, a 50-bed nursing home, and 1.3 physicians per 10,000 population.

Based on identified need, the community, with assistance from Auburn University at Montgomery School of Nursing, developed and submitted a proposal that was funded by the W. K. Kellogg Foundation. From the inception of the proposal, the philosophy was to initiate a community-based project. *Community based* means that problem identification, plans, intervention and evaluation are shared with the community. Therefore, the School of Nursing established an advisory committee composed of several representatives from the target area, as well as representatives from local and state agencies, politicians, and ministers. This advisory committee developed the project named by the community as the Rural Elderly Enhancement Program.

DESCRIPTION OF REEP SERVICES

Promoting Health and Independence. A goal of the program is to develop a model for promoting the health and independence of the elderly by linking them with human and material resources. In the model that has emerged during the past two years, the three REEP nurses in the two counties are practicing in a manner similar to that of the community health nurses who were at one time hired by a town or a county. The nurses are not tied to a fee-for-service or to a reimbursement mechanism, and so can respond to any older client's need in a timely and efficient manner. Health care and service professionals from home health care agencies, public health departments, community health centers, departments of human resources, and private practice, as well as family members and citizens, refer clients to the nurses for assessments.

In-Home Assessment. The nurses complete in-home assessments using an elderly assessment tool to gather physical, psychological, socioeconomic, and environmental data. Based on assessment data, the nurses identify appropriate resources and make referrals to meet identified needs. The nurses' activities related to coordination and advocacy involve facilitating service delivery on behalf of the client, communicating with health and human service providers, promoting assertive client communication, and guiding the client toward the use of appropriate community resources.

Follow-up assessments are completed by the nurses according to a rotation schedule based on client need. The nurses, acting as liaisons between service providers and between the client and service agencies, have decreased service duplication, increased interagency cooperation, and prevented serious illnesses by facilitating early client intervention.

The nurses work as partners with the two community development coordinators, who assist in identifying resources and organizing and sustaining volunteer coalitions. With guidance from the coordinators, the communities have responded to the special needs of the elderly by volunteering to provide services.

REEP VOLUNTEER COMPONENT

Volunteers have a vital role in REEP. Anyone with the desire to be of service to the elderly in the community can become a member of one of the volunteer coalitions. These groups are organized for various tasks, such as providing transportation, friendly visiting, assisting in housing repair or respite services, tending to correspondence, or taking care of yard work and other chores for the elderly or disabled in the community. Rewards for volunteering are:

- opportunity for skill development and job preparation;
- recognition and service to the community;
- creating new friendships; and
- letters of recommendation for employment and college scholarships.

REEP COALITIONS

The volunteers have formed groups known as coalitions, which work to enhance the quality of living for elderly residents by accepting referrals and providing services to those with special needs. The following is a list of the coalitions and their specific purposes.

Helping Hand Coalitions. Helping hand/friendly visiting coalitions provide companion, homemaker, respite, personal care, and transportation services. The committees of the homemaker service provide help with cleaning, cooking, washing, and grocery shopping to those elderly unable to do so. Respite workers provide relief for those individuals confined because of the constant care they must give an ill elderly relative. Friendly visitors visit those elderly who are isolated in order to prevent fear, boredom, and depression. Transportation is provided to elderly individuals to maintain an acceptable level of functioning. The goal of these groups is to assist those elderly who do not qualify for Medicaid waiver services and do not have sufficient income to hire persons to help with the activities of daily living.

Chore Service Coalition. Volunteers for this coalition perform such chores as yard work for those elderly who can't manage these chores alone.

Education Coalitions. After receiving health promotion training, the education coalitions provide training for the elderly and their families to improve the elderly's quality of life. One education coalition started a caregiver's support group whose membership includes adolescent boys who live with elderly families and at times are primary caregivers. The coalition identified these boys and observed that many were emotionally disturbed and none had a male figure in their lives. Consequently, the coalition initiated some intergenerational sharing with men in the coalition who are assisting the boys to become involved in community activities and employment. Some of the boys have volunteered for the housing coalition.

Housing Coalitions. Housing rehabilitation that includes ramps, porches, rails and roofs, and structural repair is done for the elderly meeting poverty guidelines. The work of private contractors is augmented by the volunteer housing coalition.

The housing coalitions have repaired 40 homes, and 120 volunteers have spent over 600 hours building ramps, steps, rails, and porches, and repairing structural damage to make homes safer for the elderly. Boy Scouts have worked with adults to complete repairs, and the vocational department of one of the county high schools, under the leadership of a retired vocational instructor, built steps and ramps at school and installed them at the homes of the elderly. The students benefited both by the practical training in construction and by becoming aware of the special needs of the elderly. Because of their work with this project, the high school vocational group received a state service award.

Fund-Raising Coalitions. The purpose of this type of coalition is to solicit funds to help defray the high cost of medical care for those elderly lacking the income and resources to maintain their medical care. The fund-raising coalitions include energetic individuals who have sold donuts, solicited donations, organized wrestling matches, and conducted raffles to raise money for such projects as buying medication and heating oil for needy elderly, and installing pipe to hook up the homes of elderly to the public water system.

Leadership Training. The goal of the REEP staff is to strengthen the community coalitions so they can continue to function when the project ends. Therefore leadership training is provided in such areas as organizing, advocacy, fund-raising, conducting meetings, strategic planning, communication, and management. Leaders have emerged from the groups who are assuming more responsibility for calling meetings, developing plans, and coordinating day-to-day operations. Coalition members are helping recruit and train volunteers and are assisting with project evaluation.

Community Health Education and Training. Another service provided by the project is community education for the elderly to improve health and quality of life. The education coordinator designs and implements training based on the needs identified by assessments. Training has included such health topics as chronic disease, nutrition, exercise, stress, and safety, as well as topics related to activities of living, such as preparing a will, managing a budget, and identifying community resources. The education coordinator also trains indigenous persons as advocates and educators for the elderly and their caregivers in the community.

The nurses and education coordinator, in cooperation with the public health department, train and certify home health aides. This is a popular activity because it targets low-income residents, and is taught in the community at a time convenient for the students. Home health agencies are eager to hire these graduates, and so all who want work are employed. Many graduates serve as volunteers for the REEP project or are caregivers for family members.

On-The-Job Training. On-the-job training is provided at the housing and water construction sites. The low-income residents who graduate from the training are employed in the target area and surrounding counties to work in construction. As a result of this training and the home health aide training, 150 people from the area are employed.

Infrastructure Improvement. Another activity of this project is infrastructure improvement, which includes housing, water, and transportation. At first this activity was not included in the project, but the community had asked grant developers how it was possible for the elderly to remain independent if they must carry water, their homes are falling down, and they had no means of transportation. There was no potable water in the eastern half of one county, and people had unsafe wells or carried water from creeks or neighbor's homes. Through a cooperative effort of state and local government and a private funding agency, a water system was built to serve 250 families.

Transportation. In cooperation with the state highway department, buses and vans were purchased and transportation routes were established to take people to the store and medical and social service providers.

FINANCIAL COMPONENT

REEP, which is a $3 million, 3-year project, is funded by a $1.4 million grant from the W. K. Kellogg Foundation and by funds and in-kind support from public and private agencies. Even though managing this program is at times difficult because of the number of agencies involved, these agencies were included so they would feel ownership and be more likely to continue activities after the funding period ended.

The Alabama Department of Human Resources supervises the activities of the two community development coordinators and pays over half of their salaries in addition to providing office space and supplies. The Tuskegee Area Health Education Commission supervises the activities of the education coordinator and contributes funds for instruction and travel. Wil-Low Non-Profit Housing Corporation, a local organization, provides staff to coordinate housing rehabilitation activities.

Nursing personnel from the county public health departments contribute clinical supervision for the home health aide trainees. Auburn University at Montgomery provides space, equipment and supplies, and half of the two nurses' salaries.

There is no charge for REEP services, and anyone age 60 or older who lives in Lowndes or Wilcox counties is eligible for services. There also are no charges for the continuing education classes and training courses.

EVALUATION OF PROGRAM

Client Profile. A progress report of the first two years of service has profiled the clientele as 640 elderly residents, 69% of whom are female and 94% black. The majority (70%) have annual incomes of less than

$5,000. Black women living alone have an average income of $3,800 per year. Sixty percent have educational levels of less than seventh grade.

The most frequently diagnosed chronic diseases are arthritis, hypertension, cardiac problems, and diabetes. A significant number of the clients reported that the pain related to the arthritis limits their activity. Many of their diets, which are high in fat, salt, and sugar, contribute to the onset and/or inability to stabilize chronic diseases. Diets also often are deficient in protein, vitamins, and minerals. Lack of money to buy food is the reason many elderly do not eat properly.

Greatest Need. The most urgent concern of these folks is housing rehabilitation. Sixty percent have housing safety problems related to rotting roofs, porches, and steps, while 40% do not have adequate plumbing or hot water.

REPLICATION OF PROGRAM

Replication of the REEP project will depend on funding for the registered nurses who are the core of this project. Of course, funding is a problem for all nurse-managed community projects because there is limited third-party payment for nurses. Parts of the project, such as the training and use of indigenous persons to serve as advocates for the elderly and their caregivers, can be replicated if an agency, such as a department of human resources or a public health department, would sponsor the activity. The model for recruiting, training, and organizing community volunteer coalitions could be replicated if an agency would provide an advisor. In this program, the Department of Human Resources provides the community development coordinators, who stimulate and maintain the activities of the coalitions.

REFERENCES AND RESOURCES

For further information, contact:

Dr. Sharon Farley, Director
Rural Elderly Enhancement Program
Auburn University at Montgomery
Montgomery, AL 36193-0401
(205) 271-9663

8

A Social Model for Community-Based In-Home Services for the Profoundly Rural Elderly
Cheyenne, Wyoming

with MARGARET A. AUKER

The Wyoming Community-Based In-Home Services Program (CBIHS) operates under the auspices of the Wyoming Commission on Aging (The Office of Aging Administration state unit). Wyoming is a profoundly rural state with sparse professional and community resources and a widely dispersed elderly population. This Rural Social Case Management model relies on paraprofessional case managers, who operate under the direction of program directors usually based in multipurpose senior centers. Their role is to assess need, develop care plans, broker/purchase in-home care, monitor, and follow up on clients and services.

PHILOSOPHY OF THE
RURAL-SOCIAL MODEL

Wyoming is the epitome of the word "rural," with only 475,000 people residing in its 97,914 square miles. Rural in this large geographic area means traveling miles for shopping, meetings, and medical services, and residents are isolated during the long winter months. Wyoming also was faced with a less-than-favorable economic status because of a bust in a once booming energy enterprise. A third problem was a shortage of professionals in fields of social work and medical care.

Flexible and Adaptive. The above factors became the innovating incentives in developing a program to serve a population continually facing the challenges presented by its geography and energy-agricultural-based economy. The state endeavored to develop a program that was flexible and adaptive, thus relying heavily on nonprofessional personnel, especially in the area of case management. It was necessary to adapt the medical-model concept of community-based in-home care to fit the local conditions.

Paraprofessional Caregivers. A key component in Wyoming's rural-social model is the cooperative relationship among paraprofessional case managers, primary care providers, and members of other private and voluntary sectors within a community in the delivery and monitoring of services. The program's accountability is based on total client involvement in making choices and evaluating outcomes and in paying their fair share of services.

HISTORY OF DEVELOPMENT
OF THE CBIHS PROGRAM

With funding provided as a result of Title III-B of the Older Americans Act, Wyoming's CBIHS program was established in 1985 as a pilot program with four Wyoming counties to develop in-home services for older persons over the age of 60 at risk of going into a nursing home prematurely. In 1987, the Commission on Aging appropriated $150,000 from State General Funds to designate the project as demonstration status for 10 counties. In 1988, 21 counties, including the Wind River Indian Reservation, received grants to fill the gaps in the comprehensive service system for the population of older persons "at risk" of premature institutional care. The Wyoming state legislature, in 1989, appropriated $300,000 to the Commission on Aging for the development of community-based/in-home services on a statewide basis. Today the program is at work in 23 counties, including the Wind River Reservation.

In 1987, the Wyoming Commission on Aging developed and implemented a quality assurance process that revolves around an instrument of standards for the three major areas of program quality: structural, process, and outcomes standards.

Pilot Projects. The program has grown from four pilot projects in 1985 to 23 county-based projects, serving over 1,400 frail elderly in fiscal year 1990. The major goals and objectives of these community programs are directed at enabling the elderly, especially the frail elderly, to remain at home and minimize their chance for premature institutionalization.

The clients themselves and the services they need to help maintain their independence, living in their own homes or apartments, are the major focus of the program.

ARRAY OF SERVICES

The community-based programs are administered under the auspices of senior centers, except for one hospital-based site. The program places a case manager in each county to help older persons and their families determine what types of services they need and at what time they are needed during the day and week. Case managers play a dual role in that they are responsible for assessments of need, identifying and planning the types and frequency of services, and monitoring service while simultaneously serving as "gatekeepers" of scarce resources to allow care money to go as far as possible in adequately meeting the needs of clients.

Each county program, through the board of directors of the designated private-nonprofit senior center or hospital provider, decides which services will be made available within the community. This flexibility allows the limited resources to fill the gaps in the community and complement, not duplicate, services that are already available. Caps are set by each county to best meet the needs of the older persons residing in each community.

Comprehensive Client Assessment. A comprehensive client assessment is completed by the case manager, the client, and family members, all of whom decide jointly what will work best for the client.

Specific services provided are adult day care, case management, home health aide, homemaker assistance, hospice care, and respite care.

Overall leadership is provided by the Wyoming Commission on Aging, which adopts rules and regulations governing the services. Figure 8.1 illustrates the delivery of services within the social model for community-based in-home services for the profoundly rural elderly.

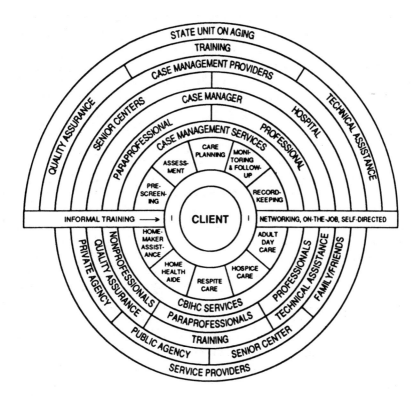

Figure 8.1. A Social Model for Community-Based In-Home Services for the Profoundly Rural Elderly.

SOURCE: Reprinted with permission of the Wyoming Commission on Aging, October 1989.

Duties for care providers and services include:

Homemaker. Homemaker duties include light housekeeping, meal preparation, and shopping assistance.

Home Health Aide. Home health aides provide personal care services such as bathing, shampooing, and nail clipping.

Adult Day Care. Day care services are provided in a congregate setting and usually one meal and a snack are provided, along with activities of interest to the participants.

Respite Care. Respite is provided to help the primary care provider get a well-deserved break from the care-taking activities. A respite care provider can come into the home to relieve the primary care provider; adult day services are available; or respite care can be arranged when another service provider is in the home and able to provide such care in addition to his or her other responsibilities.

Hospice Care. Hospice services are provided for the terminally ill.

Training Workshops. The Wyoming Commission on Aging has developed training workshops for CBIHS case managers, project directors, and bookkeepers that focus on the purposes and processes of case management, community resources, and issues of aging. Such workshops are meant to complement or supplement academic and work experiences of those involved in order that they carry out expected duties and work closely with nursing and social work professionals to determine the availability of resources and services in their communities and to match clients with appropriate resources. Recently, a quality assurance component has been added to the case management curriculum.

FINANCIAL COMPONENT OF
THE CBIHS PROGRAM

State and Federal Sharing. Though the 1985 start-up funding came from Title III-B of the Older Americans Act, today only 4% of the program's budget is provided by Title III-D. Funding has shifted and expanded, with 52% allocated from the Wyoming State Legislature, 28% from client cost-sharing, and 16% from local communities.

Clients/Families. Since 1985, on a statewide basis, the clients or their families have paid up to one-third of the total cost of the program. The cost for the services is discussed with the client and his or her family during the care planning stage. Most clients feel strongly about paying their fair share for the services received because they realize that without these services they would be paying for nursing home care. If it is determined that the client cannot afford these services, the services will be provided at no cost to the client.

Medicaid Waiver. Wyoming does not participate in the Medicaid Waiver program for home- and community-based services. However, it is expected that the waiver will be adopted by January 1991, adding a new funding alternative and/or supplement. During the program's first year, program funding was provided as follows: state general funds, $150,000; local funds from cities and counties, $12,623.06; other funds from the Commission on Aging, $9,814.39; and clients or family members, \$86,745.01—for a total cost of \$261,191.46. The average cost per client for that year was \$743.17, and the average total cost per month, \$39.43. Of the 552 persons served, 157 individuals were considered Medicaid eligible. If these individuals would have been placed in institutional care, the average cost per month to the state would have been \$900 (or \$1,695,600 for the year). By 1988 the total budget expanded to \$332,398.44 and served 930 people in 10 counties, with an estimated savings of \$1,243,300. With expanded services, the 1989 estimated savings to the State of Wyoming totaled \$2,096,384.78.

EVALUATION

The Commission on Aging has implemented a program to assure that the in-home services project is doing what it was designed to do. A review team completes an on-site assessment with each county project on a quarterly basis. The team meets with the senior center project director, the case manager, and a random sample of clients to determine the quality and progress of the program.

The clients candidly share their concerns and satisfaction with services received under the community-based, in-home services program. This is a valuable report that helps solve problems and determine whether the program is meeting the goal of assisting older persons to stay in their homes.

Quality Assurance. In order to expedite the development of the quality assurance process and to improve its monitoring mechanisms, the Commission on Aging applied for and received an Administration on Aging discretionary grant in 1988. Four objectives were realized for this project:

1. The first primary objective in the grant included statistical analysis of the quality assurance instrument in order to determine its content validity and interrater reliability. Content validity was assessed by reviewing current literature and Wyoming Commission on Aging documents and by conducting informal interviews with commission personnel. Interrater reliability was determined by computing Pearson correlations on data obtained from 12 site assessments.

2. A second objective involved the further development of an existing training program to provide information and technical assistance to the

    local grantees regarding the improvement of quality assurance activities through monitoring and documentation procedures.

3. The third primary objective was to complete quarterly on-site assessments in 20 counties involved in the project.

4. The fourth objective involved the commission's dissemination and utilization activities in providing presentations; workshops; training intensives; video education programs; and general-information-sharing programs regarding the written analysis of the quality assurance instrument, the training products, and the final results of this federal discretionary project, at a state, regional, and national basis over the 17-month duration of the project.

Through the joint efforts of the Wyoming Commission on Aging staff, an independent consultant to this project, and a postdoctoral fellow from the Gerontological Society of America, an evaluation was made of the results of the statistical analysis of the instrument, the training products, and on-site assessment process. Recommendations then were made regarding the future direction of the quality assurance program for rural in-home care.

Validity. Viewed from the perspective of "locality relevance" (e.g., measuring the quality of programs and services for the rural elderly on the basis of their ability to meet local needs), the assessment instrument possesses content validity. In other words, it does reflect the "standards and criteria" that have been adopted and incorporated into the case management training curriculum, and does measure those concepts that undergrid the social model and are translated into knowledge, skills, and abilities via case management training.

Reliability. As for the interrater reliability, 8 of the 12 statistical correlations were significant and ranged from 0.26 to 0.77; in addition, at least one of the two correlations per pairing was significant. These results suggested that there is a positive relationship between each of the paired raters, although some pairings are stronger than others. Even though not all of the correlations were significant, the findings are encouraging, especially since the correlations for the two outside raters were two of the strongest overall.

The quality assurance assessment process and the social model for community-based in-home care of which it is a part can be adapted easily to other rural environments.

In 1989, the Wyoming Community-Based, In-Home Services Program for the Elderly saved the state of Wyoming 1.2 million dollars that would have had to be paid for unnecessary nursing home care. During that year, the project served a total of 1,200 clients, of which 681 received direct-purchased services. The average cost to the state is $385 per year, or $32 per month per client. In contrast, the average cost of nursing home care under Medicaid is $1,500 a month.

The 1989 survey showed that 25% of the individuals at risk of nursing home care have funds to fully pay for nursing home care, 45% of which have limited funds to pay for nursing home care and most of whom would exhaust their funds very quickly if they had to spend $1,500 per month. The In-Home Services Program is a cost-effective alternative to nursing home care for those persons needing some assistance in maintaining their independence.

During the fiscal year 1989, all individual and program data were tracked through the computer programs at the Commission on Aging office. Individual client data provided information for the data base and was then accessed for products that were used in planning for the 1991-92 Biennium Budget request.

REPLICATION OF THE CBIHS PROGRAM

Flexibility and coordination of resources are the keys to the replication success of CBIHS. Twenty-three counties, including the Wind River Indian Reservation, have tailored a program to serve the needs of the elderly by coordinating with a board of directors and program case manager.

Cooperative Relationship. A key component of this "social" model is the cooperative relationship among paraprofessionals, case managers, primary care providers, and members of other private and voluntary sectors within a community in delivering and monitoring of services. Inherent in the model is the program's accountability to the client and family; it acknowledges that quality of life and quality of care in home-based care is uniquely client specific. Client involvement in making choices and evaluating outcomes is elicited and relied on to the greatest extent feasible. This client involvement extends the client's role in paying for his or her fair share of services that are put in place. Client and family involvement in making choices and purchasing needed services can lead to improved coordination of services and a greater sense of responsibility for monitoring the beneficial outcomes, as well as problems, in the services delivered (Auker & Kimboko, 1989, p. 9).

RESOURCES AND REFERENCES

Auker, M. A. (1990, May). *Quality assurance for profoundly rural, paraprofessional case management services.* Paper presented at the Mid-American Congress on Aging, Kansas City, MO.

Auker, M. A., Darrah, S. J., & Kimboko, P. J. (1990, March). *Quality assurance for profoundly rural, paraprofessional case management services.* Paper presented at the annual meeting of the American Society on Aging, San Francisco, CA.

Auker, M. A., & Kimboko, P. J. (1989). *Quality assurance in rural managed in-home care: The Wyoming CBIHS Program Model.* Paper presented at the meeting of the American Society on Aging, Washington, DC.

Kimboko, P. J. (1985). *Wyoming Community-Based In-Home Services Program: Preliminary evaluation.* (Research Report, Postdoctoral Fellowship Program in Applied Gerontology of the Gerontological Society of America). Cheyenne, WY: Commission on Aging, State of Wyoming.

Kimboko, P. J. (1989). *Quality assurance for case management programs: Review and application of the CBIHS standards.* Paper presented at the workshop on quality assurance in long-term care, sponsored by the Wyoming Commission on Aging, Jackson, WY.

Kimboko, P. J. (1986). *Final evaluation report: Wyoming Community-Based In-Home Services Project, July 1985-December 1985.* (Research Report, Wyoming Commission on Aging, Cheyenne, Wyoming). Greeley, CO: MESU Associates.

Sessions, S. E., & Auker, M. A. (1990, May). Quality assurance of case management services for rural, community-based, in-home care for the elderly: Final Report. Submitted to the Administration on Aging, Department of Health and Human Services, Washington, DC.

Sharp, D. S. (1989). *An assessment instrument for measuring the quality of case management services for rural, community-based, in-home care for the elderly.* Cheyenne, WY: Commission on Aging.

State of Wyoming, Department of Labor. (1989). [Supply and demand of nurses and social workers]. Unpublished raw data.

State of Wyoming, Commission on Aging. (1988). *Quality assurance for rural in-home care: A federal coordinated discretionary grant proposal.* Cheyenne, WY: Commission of Aging, State of Wyoming.

State of Wyoming, Department of Administration and Fiscal Control, Division of Research and Statistics. (1988). *Wyoming Population and Employment Forecast Report* (10th ed.). Cheyenne, WY: Author.

State of Wyoming, Legislative Service Office. (1990). *Program evaluation: Commission on Aging.* State Audit Report. Cheyenne, WY: Commission on Aging.

State of Wyoming, Commission on Aging. (1989). *Community based in-home services for the elderly: A rural, social case management model.* Cheyenne, WY: Commission on Aging, State of Wyoming.

For further information on the Social Model for Community-Based In-Home Services for the Profoundly Rural Elderly, contact:

Deputy Director
Wyoming Commission on Aging
139 Hathaway Building
Cheyenne, WY 82022-0710
(303) 777-7986 or 1-800-442-2766

9

PASSPORT: Pre-Admission Screening System for Providing Options and Resources Today
State of Ohio

with ROBERT A. APPLEBAUM

Ohio's PASSPORT (Pre-Admission Screening System for Providing Options and Resources Today) program is designed to expand and coordinate long-term care for aged and disabled people with chronic disabilities. PASSPORT is the Ohio initiative designed to slow the growth of future state long-term spending while at the same time dramatically expanding the availability of community-based long- term care, and providing persons with long-term care needs with options whenever possible.

HISTORY OF PASSPORT

Channeling Demonstration: Ohio's participation in the National Long-Term Care Channeling Demonstration (1980-1985) was an important milestone in the development of the PASSPORT program. The Channeling Demonstration called for initiatives at two levels. At a local site (Cuyahoga County), an experimental demonstration of the provision of case management services to frail and impaired older people was designed and implemented. At the state level, participation in the Channeling Demonstration required the formation of a long-term care planning group to examine the state of long-term care service delivery in Ohio.

Ohio's Long-Term-Care Plan: The Ohio Long-Term Care Planning Group was formed in 1980 and included representatives from the following state departments and commissions: Human Services; Health, Economic and Community Development; Mental Retardation and Developmental Disabilities; Mental Health; Transportation; Rehabilitation Services; Aging; and the Office of Budget and Management.

The group's agenda consisted of three major issues: cost containment in the delivery of long-term care; quality of services provided; and the development of strategies designed to improve cooperative planning across those state agencies responsible for long-term care programs.

In early 1981, by executive order of the governor, the group was reorganized, with no change in membership, and renamed the Ohio Long-Term Care Council. This group proposed a Preliminary Plan for Long-Term Care in Ohio that called for linking nursing home pre-admission screening of applicants to home care alternatives. The decision to emphasize this component, named PASS (Pre-Admission Screening System), was the initial effort in the subsequent development of PASSPORT.

By May 1983, PASS had become transformed into PASSPORT (Pre-Admission Screening System for Providing Options and Resources Today). The program was initiated in two demonstration sites, encompassing nine counties in central and southwestern Ohio. In 1986, the program expanded into two additional regions of the state, Akron (Summit and Portege counties) and Cincinnati (Hamilton County). In July 1990, the state received an expanded waiver for the program. Current plans call for statewide implementation by January 1991. The expanded waiver includes a similar service package but expands considerably the income eligibility (from $365 to $725 per month) for entry into the program.

PASSPORT PROGRAM DESCRIPTION

Administration. Prior to 1988, PASSPORT was jointly administered by the Ohio Department of Human Services (the state Medicaid agency) and the Ohio Department on Aging (The State Unit on Aging). The Department of Human Services was responsible for administering the PASS, or nursing home pre-admission screening, portion of the program and was the primary gatekeeper for the program, providing both eligibility determinations and functional assessment for program applicants. The Department of Aging was responsible for administering the PORT, or home care services, aspect of the program. Today the Ohio Department on Aging is the principal administrative agency.

Individuals who are assessed by PASSPORT as having a nursing-home-level-of-care need, but who, in the judgment of the assessment team and the applicant's physician, can safely stay at home at a lower public cost and who voluntarily choose home care are enrolled in the Home Care Program. The PASSPORT Home Care Program is sometimes referred to as the "PORT" half of PASSPORT.

Case Management. In the PASSPORT Home Care Program, each enrolled client has an assigned case manager, who has special authority to order and pay for appropriate in-home services to substitute for nursing home care. Thus the PASSPORT case manager arranges for the most appropriate and efficient mix of formal services to complement the informal services provided by family caregivers. These formal services must cost less, on average, than the Medicaid cost of nursing home care. For a PASSPORT Home Care Program service plan to be considered viable it must be approved by the case manager, client, client's family caregivers, and client's physician.

Case management is clearly a key component to the PASSPORT intervention. The case manager's responsibility is to make sense of a complex, fragmented service system, ensuring adequate linkage of client needs and services. It is the responsibility of the case manager to continually monitor the client's condition and the services provided.

PASSPORT's ARRAY OF SERVICES

PASSPORT provides a large array of services: adult day care, case management, durable medical equipment, home health aide, home-delivered meals, homemaker, medical supplies, minor home modifications, physical therapy, respite care, and skilled nursing. Chore services, counseling/social work, occupational therapy, and speech therapy are new services that were added to the program by the 1990 waiver.

The program is operated at the local level by the regional area agency (except in one region of the state that uses a private not-for-profit agency to administer PASSPORT). At the local delivery system the following functions are performed:

Screening/Intake/Eligibility Determination. The primary referral sources for PASSPORT clients are nursing homes, county departments of human services, public health nurses, hospitals, families, and community agencies. Intake screening may occur over the telephone or in person and involves identifying those persons who are currently Medicaid eligible or those seeking Medicaid reimbursement for institutional care. After passing the intake screen, applicants are immediately scheduled for a comprehensive assessment.

Assessment. PASSPORT assessment teams consisting of a nurse and social worker are either hospital based or community based. In some cases, hospitals use their own staff to assess patients just prior to discharge on a subcontractual basis or request a community-based team to assess patients within the hospital.

The assessment instrument selected for PASSPORT is a standardized, comprehensive approach to determine an individual's long-term care needs. Based on the data gathered during the assessment, the assessor will design a level of care, determine the likelihood of Medicaid eligibility, and analyze options available to individuals to meet their care needs.

Members of the assessment team identify and discuss alternatives for long-term care with the individual and, if available, members of their informal network. The alternatives for Medicaid clients are primarily a function of the level of care assignment. Medicaid clients assigned an intermediate or skilled level of need have a choice of either 2176 home-care services supervised by a case manager or nursing home placement.

Medicaid clients whose care needs are determined to be inappropriate for institutional care are offered assistance in developing a care plan that consists of traditionally funded home care services. Case management, a 2176 waiver-funded service, is not extended to this group of clients. A care plan is developed for those clients determined to be eligible for the program.

Care Planning. Care planning is a process of identifying and arranging for the delivery of services designed to meet the individual's health, psychological, and social needs in order to remain in the community. The care plan is based on data gathered in the comprehensive assessment. Initial development of the care plan is carried out by the assessment team, which specifies the name of each service to be delivered, the frequency and amount of service, and an estimate of cost that is not to exceed 60% of annual Medicaid costs for institutional care in the service area.

Case managers project the cost of client care over a 6-month care planning period to ensure that costs are kept beneath the cap. The case manager maintains authority over the amount, scope, and duration of services authorized and paid by the agency. Services are performed by providers under contract at a defined cost per unit of service. The case manager may develop a new 6-month care plan for a currently enrolled client as a result of a routine 6-month assessment, or at any time an event-based reassessment warrants a new care plan.

Following the completion of the care plan, case managers begin the service ordering process. Ongoing monitoring assures that services are delivered and meet client needs. Periodic reassessment to adjust the care plan to changing client needs is also necessary.

PASSPORT's FINANCIAL COMPONENT

The majority of services for program clients are purchased through the Medicaid Waiver but funding provided by Medicare, Social Services Block Grant, and the Older Americans Act is also used.

Clients who qualify for PASSPORT can receive waiver services, including case management, within the PASSPORT overall cost cap limits and health and safety considerations.

Service-Cost Distribution. Service costs for the PASSPORT Program are distributed as follows: home health nursing, 35%; homemaker/chore, 18%; respite, 17%; adult day dare, 8%; home-delivered meals, 7%; case management, 7%; equipment and supplies, 5%; physical, occupational, and speech therapies, 1%; transportation, 1%; and counseling/social work, 1%. Approximately 2 to 4% of clients in the PASSPORT program receive adult day care services. Adult day services are frequently provided for respite care if caregivers must work outside the home to support the client and themselves. These clients might otherwise require nursing home placement due to the absence of a caregiver 6 to 8 hours per day.

Cost Effectiveness. The addition of new services and the expansion of PASSPORT statewide must meet the Health Care Financing Administration's test of cost effectiveness. Since Ohio's Department of Aging has agreed to be at cost risk that the average cost of PASSPORT

Home Care will not exceed 60% of the net Medicaid cost of nursing home care, cost effectiveness is easy to demonstrate. The expansion of Medicaid eligibility is a new Medicaid program option that cannot be denied if Ohio can demonstrate cost effectiveness and a reduction in the historic trend of nursing home bed growth.

EVALUATION OF PASSPORT

The Quality Assurance System: To develop a quality assurance system for PASSPORT, the Department of Aging, in conjunction with the Scripps Gerontology Center, Miami University, received a grant from the Administration on Aging. The philosophy of the project was that the responsibility and effort to ensure quality must be integrated throughout the organization to include every service-specific activity. Thus the overall responsibility for ensuring quality rests within the organization, even though outside monitors and review are often mandated. Four practice principles are considered in the model:

1. Staff across all levels of the agency must be involved in the quality assurance process.
2. Staff must have specific quality assurance responsibilities and time set aside to complete them.
3. Outside consultants may be helpful in designing and implementing quality assurance activities, but these activities are the ultimate responsibility of staff.
4. Agency administration staff as well as each level of the organization with the service system must have a strong commitment to quality and quality assurance.

The Ohio Quality Assurance was an initial response to the growing need among case management and home care agencies for reliable quality assurance methods. The intent of the project was to establish a model quality assurance system for case-managed, in-home care, and a range of standards and strategies that could be useful both within and beyond Ohio's PASSPORT program (Phillips, Applebaum, Atchley, & McGinnis, 1989).

Projections. Ohio's Department of Aging's designated PASSPORT local administrative agencies will perform 18,000 initial assessments in state fiscal year (SFY) 1990 and 43,700 assessments in SFY 1991,

SFY 1992, and SFY 1993. PASSPORT will be assessing individuals who are required to be assessed by PASSPORT to obtain a Medicaid level of care determination for possible admission to a Medicaid nursing home bed, and individuals of any income who are considering nursing home placement but would like to remain at home, if possible.

About 10% of all the individuals assessed each month will be enrolled in the PASSPORT Home Care program, 70% will enter nursing homes, and 20% will be helped in selecting other alternatives to nursing home placement that are appropriate to those individual's needs and incomes. In any given month, about 5% of the clients enrolled in the PASSPORT Home Care program leave the program, many due to death.

EXPANSION OF PASSPORT

The Ohio legislature recently approved expansion of the PASSPORT program, with a 57% increase for 1990 ($12.7 million) and an 88% increase for 1991 ($23.9 million). Additional funds were allocated to establish an elder care pilot program in one urban and one rural site to provide PASSPORT services to non-Medicaid-eligible persons.

Funds were also approved to develop alternative housing options for elderly persons, provide transportation to medical and social services, augment home delivered meals, and establish a home care ombudsman program.

Statewide Service System. By January 1991, PASSPORT will be a statewide service system. By June 1991, about 7,000 individuals will be receiving PASSPORT Home Care as their preferred substitute for more expensive nursing home care. It is expected by 1992 that 12,829 home care enrollees will be served at a projected average cost per client of $1,030.95 per month.

REFERENCES AND RESOURCES

Applebaum, R. A., Atchley, R. C., & Austin, C. D. (1987). *A study of Ohio's Passport Program.* With the support of the Department of Health and Human Services.
Applebaum, R. A., Atchley, S. J., McGinnis, R., & Bare, C. A. (1989). *A guide to ensuring the quality of in-home care: Final report of Ohio's Quality Assurance Project.* With the support of the Department of Health and Human Services under grant No. 90-AM-0171.

Phillips, P. D., Applebaum, R. A., & Atchley, S. J. (1989). Assuring the quality of home-delivered long-term care: The Ohio quality assurance project. *Home Health Care Services Quarterly, 10* (3/4), 45-65.

Phillips, P. D., Applebaum, R. A., Atchley, S. J., & McGinnis, R. (1989). Quality assurance strategies for home-delivered long-term care. *Quarterly Review Bulletin, 15* (5), 156-162.

For further information, contact:

Anne Harnish, Director
Ohio Department of Aging
50 West Broad Street
Columbus, OH 43266-0501
(616) 466-5500

10

The Nursing Home Without Walls
State of New York

with TARKY LOMBARDI, JR.

The Nursing Home Without Walls (NHWW) program is exactly as its name describes—a program that provides nursing home level care to patients in their own homes rather than requiring them to be institutionalized.

The NHWW provider (approved hospitals, nursing homes, and home health agencies), in collaboration with local departments of social services (LDSS), provide and coordinate a comprehensive range of health, social, and environmental services tailored to patients' individual needs and managed on a 24-hour, 7-day-a-week basis. The program makes available in patients' homes the same comprehensive long-term care that is otherwise available only in nursing homes.

PHILOSOPHY OF THE PROGRAM

The goal of NHWW is to reduce the human and fiscal costs involved in institutionalizing chronically ill persons while increasing the quality of life for individuals. The program explicitly includes a cost cap as well as an expanded set of medical and social services.

The philosophy of the program is provided by its consistency throughout the state. NHWW is designed to meet the increasing need for long-term care and simultaneously help contain the high costs to public and private payers. Patient care costs under this program have consistently been about half the cost of comparable levels of institutional care. Since the program is a substitute for long-term facility care, the need for expensive construction is reduced.

HISTORY OF DEVELOPMENT

By the mid-1970s, the increases in population most at risk, bias toward and overdependence on the institutional care system, skyrocketing costs, and patient's preference to remain at home resulted in the need for a shift in focus for better methods of providing and financing long-term care. New York State Senator Tarky Lombardi, Jr., then chairman of the New York State Senate Health Committee, was concerned by these trends, particularly the number of persons forced by the public payment system to enter institutions. Consequently, he developed the Nursing Home Without Walls concept—a humane, less costly, and flexible alternative for providing long-term care.

Pioneer in the Delivery of Long-Term Care. Senator Lombardi envisioned the Nursing Home Without Walls Program as an approach that would not only target the immediate crisis, but that would pioneer a new direction in the delivery of long-term care. He designed this alternative program to provide long-term care that was custom-tailored to the needs of the patients at home without providing extra, unnecessary services and without requiring the patient to fit into the fixed routine of an institution. The program was conceived to provide more than just traditional home care, but nursing-home-level care to patients in their homes—truly a nursing home without walls. On August 11, 1977, Senator Lombardi's legislation, Chapter 895, made New York's Nursing Home Without Walls program a reality.

Start-Up and Development. The program began in 1978 with nine pioneering providers and a state-limited capacity to serve 805 patients. The Nursing Home Without Walls program was so different and so comprehensive, and its mandate so challenging, that a lengthy start-up phase was, in many ways, inevitable.

Nursing Home Without Walls introduced a new and entirely different approach to providing care at home. The range of services, focus of care, and targeted patient groups varied significantly from traditional home health programs. Providers and local social services departments, as well as referring agencies, health professionals, and communities generally, needed time to become familiar with the unique features and potential patient benefits. Particularly difficult was learning to identify appropriate patients. Referring agencies and program staff had to learn how this new program could appropriately maintain nursing-home level patients at home within its cost limitations. It took a great deal of time and commitment to learn how this program could simultaneously fulfill its exceptional service mandate, as well as its policy and economic goals. Practical matters concerning implementation required extensive time and effort. Service contracts, policies, and procedures had to be established.

Initially, the administration viewed the program as a pilot project, limiting the number of participating providers and the total patient capacity until effectiveness could be demonstrated. Early expansion was also constrained by an initial belief on the part of some local officials and providers that their communities "already received an equivalent service" or the belief that the program would "only work in service-rich metropolitan areas."

In 1980, legislative amendments were a significant stimulus to the program, as well as its inclusion in New York's bed planning methodology for long-term care. This methodology requires that a percentage of the projected bed need be met through the development and expansion of the NHWW program as a direct alternative to the construction of facility beds. This policy helped encourage NHWW's growth throughout the state and contributed to the development of its integral role in New York's overall long-term care system.

Catastrophic Health Care Expense Program. In 1988, New York allocated $7 million to three counties to implement pilot programs with a family "cost-sharing" component. The program was designed to assist persons and families to meet the extreme cost of catastrophic illness without first requiring them to become impoverished or disabled to the point of relinquishing employment. This program was a first step for New York toward filling the gaps left by present payment systems and perhaps will lead to statewide implementation.

Discrete Home Care Services for AIDS Victims. In an effort to open access to the program to persons with AIDS, Senator Lombardi developed legislation, subsequently enacted as Chapter 622 of the Laws of 1988, that allows Nursing Home Without Walls providers to provide specialized home care for AIDS patients. Effective January 1, 1989, the amendment allows Nursing Home Without Walls providers, as part of their programs, to provide discrete AIDS home care services. Services to AIDS patients under this special initiative will not be subject to a cost cap. Providers must apply for and receive the commissioner of health's authorization to provide the AIDS home care program. Procedures for patient assessment, authorization and management of care, and the range of services, including waived services, are essentially the same as for Nursing Home Without Walls patients generally. Modifications may be made as appropriate so that the services can be oriented to the specific needs of AIDS patients, and additional services necessary for the care of such patients may be authorized for these AIDS home care programs. Applications are now being filed for special AIDS home care designation.

Response to Continuing Problems and Trends. The need to address the continuing problems and trends in long-term care has been significant in the expansion of Nursing Home Without Walls. The increased demand for long-term care, rising health care costs, high incidence of premature/inappropriate institutional placements, and patient and family preference for care at home provided strong incentives for the establishment of NHWW's service.

Nursing Home Without Walls, having demonstrated its effectiveness in responding to these problems and trends, is now firmly established as an integral part of New York State's long-term care system.

Statewide System. At the end of June 1990, 111 providers have been approved in 52 of New York's 62 counties, with a combined capacity to serve nearly 15,000 patients. Ninety-four of these providers have become operational, with a combined caseload of about 9,400 patients. In addition, applications for new programs and for the expansion of existing programs continue to be filed. It remains a state objective that NHWW be available to all New Yorkers who would prefer an alternative to long-term institutional care.

Distinguishing Features. The Nursing Home Without Walls legislation established the essential design for the program and incorporated certain features that have been instrumental to its continuing success as an alternative to institutionalization. These key features, which are largely unique to Nursing Home Without Walls and distinguishes it from traditional forms of community care, are encapsulated in Table 10.1.

Table 10.1 Distinguishing Features of the Nursing Home Without Walls Program

Selection of Providers	Participating providers must be licensed hospitals, residential health care facilities, or certified home health agencies, and be specifically approved to provide NHWW.
Partnership Between Provider & Local District	Locally, programs and patients are managed through joint involvement by NHWW providers and local social services departments.
Patient Eligibility	Patients must be medically eligible for skilled nursing or health-related facility care. Medically eligible persons are eligible for NHWW regardless of age or payer source.
Requirement for Notification & Referral	All Medicaid patients medically eligible for skilled nursing or health-related facility care must be notified of the availability of the NHWW program and, if interested, be referred for an assessment.
Comprehensive Assessments	Each patient receives a comprehensive health, social, and environmental assessment prior to admission and at least every 120 days.
Wide Gamut of Care	A broad range of services is available and Medicaid reimbursable. Over 20 discrete services are available; 13 services are required, and additional services may be provided through a federal waiver.
Case Management & Service Coordination	Each patient receives total, ongoing case management and service coordination. Professional assistance is available on a 24-hours, 7-days-a-week basis.
Cost Cap	Expenditures for patient care are capped at 75% of the average rates of payment for skilled nursing or health-related facility care within the patient's area of residence. Exceptions include care costs for residents of adult homes, which are capped at 50% of the SNF or HRF rate, and case-specific approval of expenditures of up to 100% for patients with special care needs.
Nursing Home Level Care at Home	Each patient is provided with a comprehensive, coordinated program of nursing home level care in their own home.

ARRAY OF SERVICES

A comprehensive range of service, covering nearly the entire gamut of patients' long-term care needs, is available and reimbursable throughout the program. Individual programs are required to provide at least 13 services; through a federal waiver (1915-c) to the Social Security Act, they may provide additional services that are not otherwise provided or reimbursed under Medicaid but that are essential to maintaining patients in the community.

Broad Range of Services. Nursing Home Without Walls services, which represent perhaps the broadest range of services available through a community care program, include:

Nursing	Homemaker
Physical Therapy	Housekeeper
Occupational Therapy	Respite Care*
Speech Pathology	Housing Improvement*
Audiology	Social Day Care*
Respiratory Therapy*	Moving Assistance*
Medical Social Services*	Social Transportation*
Nutritional Counseling*	Congregate Meals*
Medical Supplies	Home-Delivered Meals*
Medical Equipment	Personal Emergency
Personal Care	Response System*
Home Health Aide	

*Medicaid reimbursable through Federal Waiver

Nursing Home Without Walls in Adult Homes. Certain adult care facility (ACF) residents, whose conditions have declined, may receive NHWW services to help them remain in their home-like setting rather than be displaced to a nursing home. Legislation was designed to help assure access to appropriate services for these residents and allow for more flexible, appropriate, and efficient use of a community's health and social services resources. To be eligible for NHWW care, ACF residents must have resided in the facility for at least six months, meet the eligibility criteria for NHWW, as well as the continued stay criteria for the facility, and be able to be cared for at a cost not exceeding 50%

of the average monthly rates for skilled-nursing facility (SNF) or health related facility (HRF) care. The procedures for assessment, management, and provision of NHWW care is generally the same as for any community resident. NHWW care must be provided by a certified NHWW provider and must be coordinated with, but not duplicate, the services rendered in the ACF. The State Social Services commissioner is required to evaluate and report on the effectiveness of this measure, which started on April 1, 1988, and is slated to end March 31, 1993.

Provision of Services. Nursing Home Without Walls provides patients with a comprehensive program of long-term care. Its coordinated design forms the basic framework for all patient care and managed activities, from the initial referral to discharge. NHWW providers and local social services departments are jointly involved in the provision of care. Actual hands-on care is provided and arranged by the NHWW providers who, for Medicaid cases, are joined by local social services departments in handling certain management responsibilities.

Team Assessments. Assessments are conducted by a team made up of a nurse employed by the NHWW provider, a social worker from the LDSS, and often the patient's physician, discharge planner, and family. The assessment then becomes the basis for the patient's care plan to assure that services are properly tailored to the patient's specific needs and are provided in the most appropriate and efficient manner.

Case Management. Case management becomes the core of the program and works to eliminate fragmentation and duplication of patient services, assures continuity of services, closely monitors all aspects of patient care, observes changes in condition or unmet needs, affords the patient and family the security of after-hours and weekend services, facilitates a close and positive relationship with the patient, and assures the most appropriate and cost-effective patient care.

Care Providers. NHWW care is provided by hospitals, residential health care facilities, and certified home health agencies specifically approved to provide this long-term home health care program. The program is available to any patient who is determined medically eligible for placement in a skilled nursing or health-related (intermediate-care) facility and who, with the provision of NHWW care, could be appropriately maintained at home. Patients must have a suitable home in which to receive care, one that has been approved by the physician and arranged for by the NHWW provider.

FINANCIAL COMPONENT

Payer Source. Medicaid is the primary payer for the Nursing Home Without Walls. About 90% of the patients in the program are on Medicaid; the remaining 10% private pay or use private insurance or Medicare only.

Cost Cap. Total cost of each patient's care is capped at 75% of the average annual cost of long-term institutional care in the patient's area of residence. Exceptions include care costs for residents of adult homes, which are capped at 50% of the SNF or HRF rate, and case-specific approval of expenditures of up to 100% for patients with special care needs.

Cost Containment and Savings. The average care costs for NHWW patients have consistently been about 50% of the cost of either skilled nursing or health-related facility care. Thus by caring for patients at home instead of in institutions, NHWW continues to result in substantial Medicaid, and hence tax dollar, savings. Greater savings are achieved in the cases in which patients would otherwise be placed in hospitals or specialty care facilities that have higher costs than nursing homes.

Costs for patient care continue to be substantially below costs for comparable levels of institutional care. Statewide, the average SNF-level patient budget was about $1,509/month, or about 68.2% of the monthly cap and 51% of the cost of care in a SNF. The average HRF-level patient budget was about $848/month, or about 60.6% of the monthly cap and 45.5% of the cost for care in an HRF. These figures represent an overall average patient cost of about $1,245/month, which is 65.1% of the allowable cap and 48.8% of residential health care facility (RHCF) care for these patients.

Mode of Operation. Generally, a referral is made to the local department of social services or NHWW provider regarding a patient's interest in receiving NHWW care. A joint assessment of the patient's health, social, and environmental needs is made that forms the basis, along with the physician's orders, for the development of a summary of service requirements, monthly budget, and plan of care. If the total cost of care is within 75% of the local average cost for a comparable level of institutional care for that patient, the case may be authorized by the local social services commissioner. Costs of up to 100% of the local skilled nursing facility or health-related facility may be authorized for certain patients with special care needs. All care is provided, arranged for, and coordinated by the NHWW provider and is specifically tailored to the patient's needs.

For Medicaid cases, the local social services department monitors various aspects of the case and, when necessary, assists in obtaining authorization and/or arranging for certain services and public benefits. Complete reassessments are conducted at least every 120 days, and the physician's orders are renewed every 60 days.

State Agency Participation. State administrative responsibilities for the NHWW program are vested in the State Department of Health and Social Services.

The State Department of Health, through its Office of Health Systems Management, is responsible for Certificate of Need review and approval, certification of providers, and rate setting for Medicaid services. It also develops regulations and procedures for local program operation and administration, carries out the surveillance process, conducts program monitoring, and, each year, calculates the maximum allowable monthly expenditures for patient care (cost caps). A major portion of the department's responsibilities are carried out by its area Offices of Health Systems Management. These regional offices also serve as a bridge between the individual providers and the department.

The State Department of Social Services, through its Division of Medical Assistance, is responsible for NHWW implementation in the local social services departments, as well as certain aspects of provider implementation. This department develops regulations and administrative guidelines for patient and program management that are used by the local social services departments and the providers, and delineate the agencies' roles in providing and managing the program. The department also administers the federal waiver for NHWW. It establishes local district responsibilities with respect to the waived services, directs provider implementation of nonmandated services, and approves the providers' initial proposal and rates for these services. The State Department of Social Services also conducts program monitoring and develops guidelines for Medicaid eligibility. In addition, through the Medicaid Management Information System, the department is responsible for provider enrollment and reimbursement under Medicaid.

EVALUATION

Overview. Nursing Home Without Walls offers a humane, effective approach to the care of the chronically ill and infirm. Persons who would have been institutionalized otherwise have been cared for at home, families have remained together, and care has been provided in a more personalized and compassionate manner. The program has enabled some persons already in an institution to return home, helped prevent at-risk community residents from further deterioration and eventual placement, and afforded many the opportunity to die at home with dignity.

Nursing Home Without Walls helps meet the increasing need for long-term care and simultaneously helps contain the high costs to public and private payers. Patient care costs under this program have consistently been about half the cost of comparable levels of institutional care. Since the program is a substitute for long-term facility care, the need for expensive construction is reduced.

Following an initial period of slow growth, NHWW is now available nearly statewide.

Patient Profile. The following patient information is based on data compiled by NHWW providers during early 1988 and largely reflects provider experience during 1987 and a total caseload count of about 8,000. Ages of patients range from newborn to 104 years; 76% of the patients are 65 or older, about 55% are 75 or older, and nearly 4% are children. Most patients (76%) are female, and 61% have care needs at the skilled-nursing facility level. While most patients (54%) live with friends or relatives, 46% live alone. Home health agencies are the primary source of referral (34.1%), followed by hospitals (28.4%) and self/family (15.4%), with about 3% referred directly by RHCFs. Most discharges (44%) are to hospitals, 16% of the patients have died at home, and nearly 15% are discharged to self-care because of marked improvement. Although length of stay varies considerably, patients typically stay in the program for about one year. Many return to the program following a brief hospitalization or other temporary discharge. The first New York City patient, admitted in May 1979, remained in the program for nearly 7 years, until her death in 1986.

Although statistics are useful in providing information on the overall characteristics and experiences of patients served by the Nursing Home Without Walls program, as well as on the program's impacts, the portrayal of individual patients, their care, and the impact the program has made on them and on their families is perhaps the most meaningful method of showing the program's value. This single case illustration is an example:

> A couple in their early sixties suffered from cancer. The wife had multiple myeloma and bone tumors that caused spontaneous bone fractures. Her husband suffered from cancer of the colon and required chemotherapy twice a week. Although they wanted to remain together, they weren't sure how they could manage. While they were both in the hospital, they were referred to the Nursing Home Without Walls program and returned home to receive personal care, 12 hours a day, 7 days a week, and weekly nursing visits to monitor their physical condition. The NHWW nutritionist assisted with special diets, and a social worker provided supportive counseling. The wife also received physical therapy to strengthen her muscles and help with transferring from bed to chair. The couple was supplied with a personal emergency response system to assure immediate contact with help in an emergency. Through the coordinated services of NHWW, this husband and wife were able to remain in their home together despite the seriousness of their illnesses, until they passed away within weeks of each other.

Benefits to Patients and Families. Through NHWW, patients who would otherwise be institutionalized are provided with an entire program of long-term care, managed and carefully tailored to their needs and preferences. Patients receive constant coverage and communicate with a single source on all matters related to their care. They neither receive unnecessary services nor must fit into the routine of an institution. The program has a wide range of services to best meet the patient's needs, support strengths, and independence and, wherever possible, address the needs of family and other informal caregivers.

NHWW is able to improve the overall health and physical functioning of many patients despite the intensity and complexity of their illness and the fact that the very nature of chronic illness and disability require a major focus of the care to be maintenance oriented.

Quality of Life. Improvement to the quality of life, although difficult to measure statistically, is a very real and significant benefit of this program. Increased quality through the program comes with improvements in patient health, psychosocial status, safety and security, and, in some cases, the return of patients from nursing homes to their own homes. Families are provided with important relief from the stress of daily caregiving responsibilities.

There has been overwhelming patient and family satisfaction with the Nursing Home Without Walls program which, particularly among vulnerable long-term care patients, is of utmost importance. NHWW ultimately helps assure a workable and acceptable program for the patient, family, and community. All of the providers report high levels of patient satisfaction.

More Appropriate Use of Institutional Services. Nursing Home Without Walls promotes more appropriate use of institutional resources. By caring for patients at home who would otherwise be institutionalized, returning patients home from facilities, and enabling patients to avoid or reduce extended hospital stays, institutional care beds are available for more appropriate use for patients who are truly unable to be at home.

Provider experiences show strong evidence of the program's effect on containing hospital and other high-cost medical care use. This is a critical area for further exploration and study.

Benefit to Communities. Nursing Home Without Walls has given communities a means of providing residents with a humane long-term care program while effectively containing health care costs. NHWW has enhanced the community's continuum of care and has promoted more appropriate and cost-effective use of both its institutional and noninstitutional resources. The program also saves public dollars by providing care at half the cost of comparable levels of residential health care and by avoiding the "bricks-and-mortar" expenses otherwise required in the construction of long-term care facilities.

REPLICATION

Model for Related State and Federal Initiatives. NHWW continues to contribute to home health and long-term care policies and initiatives on both the federal and state levels.

Nursing Home Without Walls served as a model for the Home and Community-Based (Waived) Services provisions of the Omnibus Budget Reconciliation Act of 1981, in which most states now participate and that very closely follows the design and features of NHWW.

Most recently, during the 1988-89 congressional legislation, the Medicare Long Term Home Care Catastrophic Protection Act, sponsored by Representative Claude Pepper, would have established nationwide, under Medicare, a Nursing Home Without Walls program patterned after that of New York. Although Congress did not act, this proposal, based on New York's success, has helped bring the urgency of long-term care and a possible national solution to a new, important level of awareness in Washington.

Elements of the NHWW design have also been incorporated into numerous other programs in New York State. The design of this program is expected to continue to contribute to long-term and home health care policies and initiatives for years to come.

Cost Containment, Cost Savings. Cost containment benefits of the NHWW program have been significant, with costs being far less than what would otherwise be expended for institutional care. The fiscal benefits of this cost-effective program continue to save millions of taxpayer dollars.

The average cost per patient for care in the Nursing Home Without Walls program has consistently been about half of the cost of skilled nursing or health-related facility care. In cases where patients would otherwise be in acute care hospitals, rehabilitation hospitals, or other facilities with higher costs than skilled nursing or health-related facilities, the program has resulted in even greater savings.

To the extent that the program is able to improve patient functioning; help prevent accidents and deterioration; and minimize acute hospitalization, emergency room use, and other high-cost medical care utilization, its costs savings benefits are increased.

Nursing Home Without Walls also helps contain costs by providing an alternative to nursing home construction or expansion. The average cost of constructing a nursing home bed in New York State ranges to over $100,000 per bed. Since there are no construction costs involved in the NHWW program, significant capital investment is avoided each time a community meets a portion of its long-term care need by substituting NHWW for the construction of additional facility beds.

The Nursing Home Without Walls program continues to result in a substantial savings of public dollars. While the total aggregate savings to public and private payers has not been compiled, the significant fiscal benefits of appropriately substituting NHWW's care for institutional care have been well demonstrated; these savings are clear when comparing the actual monthly cost for patient care in the program with the monthly reimbursement rates for care otherwise provided in institutional settings, primarily skilled nursing and health-related facilities. This savings is also apparent when comparing total Medicaid expenditures for long-term care patients in New York State with projected aggregate expenditures if the program were unavailable. Although not finalized, current projections being prepared for submission to the federal government for purposes of statistical reporting on New York's waiver show a continuing, significant cost-change to New York as a result of the program.

CURRENT AND FUTURE ISSUES

Some of the developments, factors, and issues that are expected to have an impact on the Nursing Home Without Walls program, as well as on long-term and home health care generally, are described below. While a great deal remains uncertain, the increasing demand and trend for care at home will continue.

Health Personnel Shortage. The increasing demand for home care services will necessarily result in an increased need for adequately trained persons to provide the required care. If reliance on the institutional care system is to be reduced and home care expanded in order to meet the increases in patient and community needs, and if quality and access are to be assured, the required personnel to provide this care must be also assured.

Financing. As the population ages, demands for long-term care increase, and costs continue to rise, the question of who will pay becomes increasingly significant. Although progress continues, neither Medicare nor private health insurers truly cover the ongoing costs of long-term care. Medicaid, which does pay for long-term care, covers only those individuals with very limited income and resources. Even those who have saved and wisely invested face impoverishment should they experience a chronic or catastrophic illness that requires long-term care.

Reimbursement. Another important aspect of financing is the reimbursement methodology. If providers are to deliver quality care and the increasing needs are to be met, particularly among the more difficult and costly cases, reimbursement methodologies must be responsive to local needs and realities. The task is not easy. Conflicts and dilemmas often occur since cost-containment goals and provider/personnel payment needs are not necessarily compatible. Legislative, as well as regulatory, proposals for refinement of the reimbursement methodology are presently under consideration.

Identifying and Addressing Barriers to Access. In looking toward a future where the need for home care and alternatives to institutionalization will remain steadily on the rise, it is critical that barriers to accessing NHWW care are identified and addressed.

Areas Without a Program. While NHWW providers exist in most regions of the state, there remain 10 counties that are not served. Nearly all of these unserved areas are considering the program, and implementation of the program in all areas of New York State continues to be a fundamental policy goal.

Misunderstandings and Lack of Public Awareness. Although there is a prominent and increasing focus on providing care to patients at home, a less-than-optimal level of understanding and awareness about the Nursing Home Without Walls program and home care generally exists. Thus an undue number of patients who could be most appropriately cared for by the NHWW program, but who are unfamiliar with it, are likely channeled to (or select) an alternate home care service or an institution. Patient referral to the program, and care at home generally, is also hindered when referring professionals, family, and even patients themselves fail to recognize that the significantly impaired and those living alone can remain in their homes if provided with NHWW care and support.

Outreach and Referral. Continuing outreach, in-service training, public seminars, and community education are essential to addressing these misunderstandings. Educational efforts must continue and be directed at the overall community, as well as at key health and social services professionals who guide patients in obtaining the necessary care.

Inadequate Long-Term Care Financing. Gaps and limitations in coverage for long-term care, especially under Medicare and private insurers, present serious dilemmas and obstacles for those seeking needed service and support. The lack of adequate financing poses access problems for most persons relying on Medicare as their primary means of health insurance, and for those whose earnings and resources are above the Medicaid level but who cannot afford to finance their own care. Improved public and private financing mechanisms are crucial to promoting full access to and coverage for Nursing Home Without Walls, as well as all long-term care. A number of initiatives are currently under way in New York in order to test the effectiveness and feasibility of expanded public and private coverage for long-term and catastrophic care.

Personnel Shortage. The shortage of essential staff, especially home health aides and personal care workers, is important and particularly affects patients with unusual needs or circumstances, those living in isolated or unsafe areas, intensive/complex cases, and/or those with difficult personalities or difficult families. Adequate access to care, especially quality care, depends on maintaining adequate staff levels. Numerous measures to address this issue are being implemented and proposed.

Bureaucratic Obstacles. Perhaps the most frustrating and unjustified barriers to long-term care are those created by overly complex, cumbersome, rigid, or lengthy administrative processes. These processes usually result from the competing need to thoroughly regulate, assure quality and accountability, promote cost effectiveness, and rationally plan health care. However, minimizing adverse impacts to patient access as a result of such processes and requirements must be a priority at both state and local levels.

Design Refinements. Possibilities for enhancing effectiveness and access through refinements to the program's features and operating procedures are constantly explored. This is what gave rise to the legislative amendments and to the AIDS home care initiative described above. For example, one aspect that has been gradually refined and has been the subject of legislative deliberation is the cost cap. Over the course of the program, the cost cap has been modified to add flexibility to patient care budgeting and ultimately to patient eligibility. Although the majority of patients are appropriately maintained within the expenditure limitations, care costs for some patients exceed the cap or are projected to do so, thereby precluding admission or continued stay on the program.

Unfortunately, interpretations of the cap by referring entities are often overly rigid and do not recognize the flexibility in patient-care budgeting allowed by the statute and implemented through creative, thoughtful care planning. Given the opportunity, seriously ill patients have been stabilized, and their care costs gradually decreased so as to fall within the cost cap. This remains a crucial educational point for referral sources for the program.

Methods of increasing flexibility, however, continue to be explored for those patients who are most appropriately and efficiently cared for by the Nursing Home Without Walls program, yet whose intensive service needs and higher care costs prevent admission or continued stay. The AIDS home care legislation is precisely an outgrowth of that effort. Further flexibility is being explored so that catastrophic-level patients desiring care in the community may receive Nursing Home Without Walls care when that program is most appropriate to their needs.

CONCLUSIONS

New York's Nursing Home Without Walls program is an effective patient-oriented alternative to long-term institutionalization. It is responsive to human needs and addresses the broader economic and public policy issues in health care today. The program continues to benefit patients, families, and communities, and contributes to state and national policies and initiatives in home health and long-term care.

Because of increasing demands, rising costs and patients' preference to remain at home, NHWW will continue to be crucial to containing health care costs and meeting patient and community needs.

New York State is particularly proud of this program and the dedicated professionals who make it work. The key to NHWW's success has been its ability to improve the quality of life for persons struggling to cope with chronic illness and to meet head on the challenges of disability. Nursing Home Without Walls offers the potential to preserve and enhance lives and to improve our society.

REFERENCES AND RESOURCES

Lombardi, T., Jr. (1987-1988). Nursing Home Without Walls, *Generations, 11* (2), 21-23.
Lombardi, T., Jr., Cardillo, A., Horton, R., & Luther, C. (1988). *Nursing Home Without Walls program, A decade of quality care at home for New York's aged and disabled.* Albany: New York State Senate Health Committee.

For further information, contact:

New York Senate Health Committee
Legislative Office Building
Empire Plaza
Albany, NY 12247
(518) 455-3511

11

The Connecticut Hospice, Inc.
Branford, Connecticut

with JOHN W. ABBOTT

The purpose of hospice, a specialized health-care program for patients and families experiencing terminal illness, is to encourage the quality and comfort of existence and to enhance life for as long as it lasts. The Connecticut Hospice, Inc., the first hospice in the United States, is a medically directed, nurse-coordinated, not-for-profit program focusing on symptom control, pain management, and emotional support for the terminally ill patient and his or her family. These needs are met by the coordinated care of several disciplines. Physicians, nurses, social workers, pharmacists, clergy, artists, and volunteers, among others, work together to ease pain and suffering and to manage symptoms of terminal illnesses, whatever their origin.

PHILOSOPHY OF THE PROGRAM

The Connecticut Hospice Mission Statement. The mission statement of The Connecticut Hospice, Inc. reads as follows:

The Connecticut Hospice shall provide quality, compassionate and competent hospice care in Connecticut to patients suffering from irreversible illness, and to members of their families. Care shall be interdisciplinary in nature, allow for family decision-making and participation in care, and shall seek to enhance quality of life for as long as life lasts. With the full support of the philanthropic community, care shall also be offered commensurate with need. Home, Inpatient and Cottage Care shall serve as a clinical model for national replication through education, training and research made essential by our unique role as the founder of hospice in America.

Goals. The goals of The Connecticut Hospice are:

1. to help patients live out their days as fully and comfortably as possible;
2. to support the family as an integral part of the hospice care;
3. to enable patients to remain at home for as long as possible;
4. to provide education for health-care lay persons and professionals;
5. to enhance and supplement existing services, not duplicate them; and
6. to provide hospice care while keeping costs down.

Care. Care provided by the Connecticut Hospice is supplied by a team of paid staff and 300 volunteers. The volunteers give more than 40,000 hours of service each year. Quality hospice care requires intensive people skills, and 75% of the annual operating budget reflects this (Friedman, 1979):

> Like a tapestry woven with many different threads, care by the Connecticut Hospice is an interplay of the skills of many different professions. Within hospice home and inpatient care, physicians, nurses, pharmacists, social workers, clergy, artists, volunteers and consultants actively assist each patient and family in resolving the myriad difficulties surrounding terminal illness. It is this "team" approach—comprehensive, coordinated, palliative care without gaps or overlaps—that truly distinguishes hospice within the health care system. (Abbott, 1988, p. 45)

HISTORY OF DEVELOPMENT

In medieval times, the term "hospice" was used to describe places of comfort for travelers along the road. The use of the word to describe programs and institutions caring for the terminally ill is especially appropriate, for the modern hospice is dedicated to making the road for the dying patient as easy as possible (Friedman, 1979).

European Model. The first modern hospice, St. Christopher's, was founded in London in 1967 by Dr. Cicely Saunders, a former nurse and medical social worker who became a physician with the express purpose of looking into the problem of pain in the dying patient. St. Christopher's is a 54-bed, in-patient facility that affords dying patients the option of moving back and forth between home and institution. It was designed by Dr. Saunders to have a strong religious foundation that she sees as a cross between a hospital and a patient's home. At St. Christopher's, the unit of care is not just the patient, but also the family; the place of care is the patient's home.

Visiting hours are unlimited. Children and the patient's pet may visit. Families come at any time, and their presence adds to the vitality of caring. The health care itself is a team effort that involves all aspects of professional and paraprofessional care. Care doesn't end when the patient dies; social workers and volunteers follow the family through the bereavement process.

America's First Hospice. Hospice care in the United States developed out of a Yale University study group that was strongly influenced by St. Christopher's. Florence Wald, former dean of the Yale School of Nursing, is one of the founders, who with her husband Henry Wald conducted a feasibility study for the establishment of a hospice in the New Haven area. The group originally intended to build an inpatient facility, but as the goals of Hospice, Inc. took shape, the group determined it was most feasible to establish the home care program first and then the inpatient facility, which would serve as a backup resource for the home-care program (Abbott, 1978).

The Connecticut Hospice, Inc., began its home care program in 1974 in an old rented house in New Haven. Half a dozen nurses, some of whom were part time, and a small clerical staff were the nucleus of today's highly structured Home Care Program. The Inpatient Care Program was established in 1980 and today cares for over 1,000 patients annually. The Cottage Hospice, a five-bed house for the indigent, terminally ill (who have no home or no one to care for them at home), was established in 1988. Cottage residents number 18 to 20 each year (Yoder & Primer, 1989).

ARRAY OF HOSPICE SERVICES

The Connecticut Hospice, Inc., provides home care, inpatient care, and Cottage-care services. The inpatient program is available as a backup for home care patient/families and also meets the needs of terminally ill Connecticut patients beyond the home care service area.

Home Care. Connecticut Hospice home-care staff members make regular visits in the greater New Haven and Mid-Fairfield county areas, and are on call 24 hours a day, 7 days a week. Connecticut Hospice works in cooperation with other sectors of the health-care services system. Home health aides work under the supervision of registered nurses, who teach the disease process and medication regimen, and, most difficult of all, help the aides comprehend and deal with the reality of a terminal disease.

Admission Criteria for Home Care. The home care patient must have a progressive terminal illness, with a prognosis limited to six months or less (also determined by the patient's referring physician and in consultation with the hospice medical staff) and the consent and cooperation of the patient's referring physician. Any physician may refer patients to the Connecticut Hospice for inpatient care.

Inpatient Care. The founders of the Connecticut Hospice sought to design and construct a building uniquely adapted for hospice care. Members of a building committee spent many hours discussing what architectural features would best facilitate the application of hospice philosophy. Some of the members of the committee visited St. Christopher's Hospice in London during this process.

Admission Criteria for Inpatient Care. The inpatient must have a progressive, terminal illness, with a prognosis limited to two months or less as determined by the patient's referring physician in consultation with the hospice medical staff. There must be consent and cooperation of the patient's referring physician, including agreement to continue care of the patient after discharge if this becomes necessary, and the need for management of pain and symptoms. Consent of the patient and family is required for both home and inpatient care.

Cottage Care Services. A new dimension of hospice care is the model known as the Connecticut Hospice Cottage, which involves the establishment of a home and substitute family for the homeless patient. In the beginning, Cottage served a diverse mixture of patients, including young adults and elderly patients with AIDS, cancer, and other terminal illnesses; however, the focus soon shifted to a primary concentration on AIDS patients. The site is a small, three-bedroom, ranch-style house adjacent to the Connecticut Hospice. The regular home-care team provides intermittent, hospice, home care services to Cottage patients, although there is paid staff around the clock to provide homemaker/home-health-aide-level care and to substitute for the family. One home care nurse is assigned as the primary nurse for all five Cottage patients, and the interdisciplinary team services are provided as needed. Volunteers provide socialization, transportation, and some light housekeeping functions, but are also trained to provide hands-on patient care. Supervised by a paid staff member, a volunteer spends a 4-hour shift per week at the Cottage.

Admission Criteria for Cottage Care. Admission criteria requires patients to be at least partially ambulatory. The mix of patients at any one time determines the amount of assistance required. Special arrangements are made for family visitation, while the staff serves as the patient's surrogate family. Before the Cottage opened, the state legislature provided legislation to allow opening without licensure or regulations having been developed in advance.

The Connecticut Hospice Inpatient Building. The founding committee wanted a geographical location that would enable patients to look out on a natural setting and yet would be close to the towns and cities that defined their service area. The committee wanted an architect willing to study hospice care who would design something unique from the viewpoint of the patient. The architect chosen was Lo-Yi Chan, who volunteered to spend time at St. Christopher's in order to create an architecture of healing. He noted that hospitals are designed to cure and that they are usually designed for staff efficiency and convenience. However, the committee wanted the building to be a therapeutic environment, designed from the patient's point of view and having an at-home feeling and a place for families (Kron, 1976).

Capacity. After considerable discussion, it was agreed to build a 44-bed building that would meet the needs of extremely ill patients requiring extensive medical and nursing care. After considering several building sites, an apple orchard in Banford was chosen as the location. The site is across the street from a school and near a church.

Structure. The building consists of two single-story, V-shaped patient wings with a commons and chapel between them. The wings are attached to a two-story administrative and service spine that is marked by a long corridor, the walls of which serve as a gallery for art created by patients or staff and people in the community.

Everyone coming to the Connecticut Hospice passes by the patient wings on the way to the entrance, which opens onto an off-street parking lot. Thus the patients have a sense of "to-ing and fro-ing" and can feel part of the ongoing life of the community. Patients, families, and visitors approach the front door, which is made of oak and beautifully carved with the Tree of Life, the symbol of the Connecticut Hospice.

Everyone goes in and out the same door. Upon arrival, every patient is greeted by a nurse, who escorts the newcomer, who often has arrived by ambulance, to the room he or she will occupy.

Immediately inside the door is a small vestibule that contains the names of donors on one wall and proclamations for community observances of hospice month on the other. There is also a small telephone to be used by visitors who arrive in the middle of the night to see patients.

Two friendly, volunteer receptionists are on duty in the reception area 12 hours a day. A small, L-shaped lounge immediately inside the entrance offers a place of sanctuary to family members. A gift shop operated by an auxiliary group, Friends of The Connecticut Hospice, graces one wall; the other wall is made of solid glass, inviting (as does much of the building) the external environment to meld with the inside space.

Each of the V-shaped patient wings has a large family room with a fireplace, cozy arrangements for seating, and space for patients either on beds, all of which are mobile, or movable multiposition chairs. The tiny nurses' station is humanized and socialized by its placement in the family room, which serves as a tension-relaxing transitional space for those on their way to visit patients. A pantry, offering refrigerator, stove, microwave, and sink for anyone desiring to prepare light meals, is also located in each family room.

The building reflects a homelike atmosphere, and visiting hours are unlimited. There are no age restrictions; infants, and children are welcome, as are pets. (When one patient wanted to see her pet goats, they were brought to the patio, and a staff nurse proved to be an expert at milking goats!)

Patient Rooms. Patient rooms are arranged in a row, with corridors on either side. On one side is a greenhouse sitting room bedecked with plants maintained by patients, family members, and gardening volunteers. The greenhouse offers a solid wall of glass to the patios outside. A service corridor with offices, supply rooms, showers, medication desks, and small family room conference rooms is located on the other side of the rooms. Wide doors and hallways offer access so that bedridden patients can be moved to the family room, the commons, or to the patios.

Because of the amount of windows and skylights, there is an ample sense of light, as well as of life and growing things, which give patients a point of reference to the outside world since they can view the movement of sun, shadows, rain, and snow. Each room has a large, easily read calendar to mark the passage of time.

Ten patient rooms, five on each wing, have four beds to allow interaction of staff, patients, and families, and to create a community effect. This arrangement allows for peer support from patients experiencing similar problems, and families can give support from bed to bed. Comfortable chairs, telephones, and televisions are standard equipment. The rooms are lined with ledges for flowers and personal possessions. There are four single rooms, assignment to which is determined by medical need, such as contagion.

At the center of the two patient wings is a commons, a large room with a skylight for a ceiling, a grand piano, and space for numerous events at which artists from the community share expressions with patients and their families.

Off the commons is a tiny, circular, nondenominational chapel, with a beautiful round table and specially designed tapestries on the wall. The chapel has been the scene of weddings and christenings. Each week a remembrance service is given for patients who died the previous week. Services reflecting the major faiths are held in the commons.

Each patient wing has a patio immediately adjacent to the greenhouse corridor. Volunteers keep the patio areas alive with flowers in season. Beds are often moved onto patio areas, and families appreciate these places for visiting.

Staff Rooms. Staff needs have also been met architecturally by totally separate staff lounges, dining room, and offices. A special innovation is a tiny glass-domed, sound-proof meditation, or retreat, room. The carpet-lined retreat has no furniture except beanbags. The room was designed so staff members could have a place for free expression of emotions without the sense of disturbing others. A sign on the door requests privacy when the room is in use.

Viewing Room. Also on the second floor is a two-part viewing room. When a patient dies, the body is wheeled through the hall to the elevator, where it is brought upstairs to a preparation room. The long and narrow viewing room next door and its anteroom lounge provide opportunity for families to view the patient and accept the reality of death. A telephone is available to call families, ministers or priests, or the undertaker. Support staff is available if needed.

A simple, tiny banner next to the door indicates whether the viewing room is in use. If the banner is red, privacy is assured. Green indicates that the room may be entered.

The building opened on July 7, 1980. A common statement made by visitors is that they expected the hospice building to be depressing, but that it was cheerful instead. Many times the children from the school across the street come to visit, sometimes dressed in Halloween costumes or other seasonal finery.

The planners wanted to free the dying patient from many burdens, including those of his surroundings, so that all available energy could be used for living out one's remaining days or weeks. The goal was to make hospice a supportive place.

Primary Nursing. Every patient in the Connecticut Hospice inpatient building has a primary nurse from the moment of admission. Under the direction of patient-care managers, primary nurses immediately begin to develop a care plan outlining how the patient will be made comfortable. The plan is updated daily, and the primary nurse acts as the communicator and facilitator for the patient and family during the entire length of stay.

Patients also have associate nurses who take shifts when the primary nurse is not on duty. Medical and nursing care is available as backup for community home-care hospice programs. Staff physicians are in house daily and are on call around the clock for patient care and for patient/family/staff conferences. Medication is never administered PRN (*pro re nata* as needed), but before it is needed, in order to prevent pain and fear of pain, as well as to prevent feelings of dependency in patients who do not like to ask for relief. There is no sophisticated resuscitation equipment, only what is needed to fulfill a patient's need for living well until he dies.

Family Counseling Services. The Connecticut Hospice, Inc., offers one-time relative consultation session for family members burdened with the stress encountered in late-stage terminal illness. This service is available at the inpatient building and is open to all Connecticut residents.

Interdisciplinary Team Caring. Care of the patient and/or family begins with a visit of one hospice team member to assess how the patient and family view their situation and to understand what the patient and/or family expects of hospice as a source of help. Although the focus is on the present situation and the family's capacity to manage, it is also important to know what the patient and/or family is like under ordinary circumstances and under stress. An understanding of cultural and behavioral patterns and long-existing tensions and conflicts in a family group helps in predicting and solving problems and in developing a care plan. A view of the family's coping mechanisms enables a staff member to support or even encourage certain behaviors that may help each individual with the work ahead (Craven and Wald, 1975). After the family interview, the hospice worker reports to the interdisciplinary team, and a care plan is then designed with the patient and/or family at the core and team workers filling in the needs of the care unit.

Members of many disciplines interact with their hospice counterparts on a daily basis. Ideally, each team member channels the care and concern of his or her colleagues in the community into the hospice caregiving process. Such community interrelationships and the team roles and team member functions are presented in Figure 11.1 (Abbott, 1988, p. 42).

Community Physicians. Physicians play a unique role in that they are a repository of medical knowledge and direct the care plan within the scope of the interdisciplinary team. The inauguration of hospice care for a dying patient requires physician approval. Hospices are required to employ physicians, but only in the larger hospice programs are such professionals employed on a full-time basis. Hospice physicians accept or reject patients, direct pain and symptom management, and work with members of all the disciplines to revise and update the continuously changing patient/family-care plan. Community physicians maintain primary patient relationships except when a hospice inpatient service staffs its own physicians (Abbott, 1988).

Nursing Care. Nursing care is essential since patients enter hospice care with a wide variety of symptoms. The hospice nurse makes regularly scheduled home visits, the frequency and length of which are determined by the patient's condition. Nurses are available 24 hours a day, 7 days a week for house calls. For inpatient settings, the Connecticut public health code requires a 1:3 staff ratio around the clock, with one registered nurse for every six patients (Abbott, 1988).

Clergy Services. A pastoral care person is a member of the interdisciplinary team as a hospice employee or volunteer. In addition, the hospice director attempts to involve community clergy of their own parishioners (Abbott, 1988).

Community Social Workers. Hospice social workers provide counseling and assist patients and their families with matters involving family decision-making, children, and special problems, such as alcoholism, AIDS, and marital stress. Patients are frequently referred to a hospice by a hospital or agency setting (Abbott, 1988).

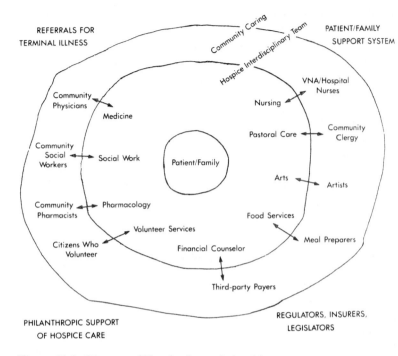

Figure 11.1. Diagram of Hospice Interrelationship.

SOURCE: Reprinted with permission as published in *Hospice Resource Manual for Local Churches*, edited by John W. Abbott. Copyright 1988, The Pilgrim Press, New York.

Community Pharmacists. A vital part of hospice care is the use of pharmacological expertise for pain and symptom management. An active, interested, community pharmacist provides helpful and efficient medications for carrying out the principles of hospice care (Abbott 1988).

Food Services. Many hospice patients who find eating very difficult because of their illness find new interest in food as a result of meal planning that aesthetically and artistically combines taste, nutrition, and palatability (Abbott, 1988).

Volunteer Services. Hospice volunteers fulfill essential roles in enlarging the options open to families and patients as well as in supportive and administrative functions. Hospice care is dependent upon dedicated volunteers who specifically choose to work in hospice. It is suggested that each volunteer have a specific job description and be a team member in a built-in network of programmatic and administrative functions (Abbott, 1988).

Volunteers augment the work of paid staff in a wide range of activities. Carefully trained in their specialties, they provide direct patient care or support that might include reading or perhaps just "actively" listening. Volunteers bolster the pastoral, arts, and bereavement departments and are drivers, barbers, retired nurses, or gardeners; they are frontline people who work behind the scenes to increase the quality of life of the patient and/or family (Fisher, 1989).

Financial Counselors. Trying to understand the intricacies of insurance coverage, Medicare, Blue Cross, and other third-party payers can be confusing. A knowledgeable financial counselor can assist patients and/their families in discovering and coordinating resources and working through financial problems (Abbott, 1988).

Artists. The arts can be a source of fulfillment in the quest of patients/families for quality of life. The hospice arts programs use musicians, graphic artists, metalsmiths, writers, movement specialists, and many other people from artistic disciplines (Abbott, 1988).

The Connecticut Hospice program gave the Reverend Sally Bailey, singer, teacher, and chaplain, the assignment to design and implement a model program in the arts for patients, families, and staff. Reverend Bailey believes that the arts are the regeneration of body, emotions, and spirit: The "whole person" is touched when one engages in an art form. The arts enable people to find meaning for their lives, to become reconnected to their spiritual roots, and the source of life, and to overcome the fragmentation in their lives. Bailey thus has incorporated the arts into the interdisciplinary scope of hospice benefits for patients and families, as well as caregivers (Bailey, 1987).

Interdisciplinary Team Functions. The physician, nurse, and pharmacist are important team members in evaluating pain and treating it pharmacologically. Artists, social workers, clergy, and nurses, as well as professional and lay volunteers, work with psychological and spiritual pain. In addition, consultants in several fields of health care complement the efforts of the medical and nursing staffs. The health care team members meet together regularly to plan and work on hospice care, developing a sense of profound trust in one another. Each discipline serves as an advocate for other disciplines so that team members can enhance the total care of the patients. Care plans are discussed confidentially for current patient, new patients admissions are considered, and changes in a patient's condition since the last team meeting are reported (Abbott, 1988).

Care Plan. The care plan must be creative, innovative, and flexible in order to respond to the constantly changing challenges of terminal illness. Some symptoms can be relieved by simple measures, such as massage, repositioning, relaxation techniques, and distraction through arts and other activities. Yet medications are often crucial in alleviating physical discomfort. An important principle in the hospice approach is that drug dosages are carefully adjusted to each patient's physical makeup to assure pain relief without a loss of alertness. The hospice goal is to control symptoms while maintaining optimum functioning and to provide relief from pain before it occurs.

The hospice interdisciplinary team is completely antithetical to a traditional medical model in which the physician is in charge of caring for the patient while members of other disciplines take orders. Rather, it is democratic, with the patient at the center.

Bereavement Care. The hospice movement demonstrates the importance of bereavement follow-up for family members. A volunteer bereavement team provides individualized care for up to a year following a patient's death. Team members have studied how best to help families with the process of grieving, and some members have been a part of hospice for many years.

Care may take the form of home visits to families, especially when there are small children, unusual problems confront survivors. Families receive periodic telephone calls whereby hospice staff inquire how things are going. Cards are sent periodically following the death of a patient. In addition, regular bereavement group meetings are held for family members. Once a year, a memorial service is held for those who died during that year.

Education, Training, and Research. The Connecticut Hospice has always had a multimission: to provide the best possible clinical care for patients and families, offer education and training, conduct research; and understand how the principles and practices of hospice may be replicated elsewhere. As a result, in 1978, the Connecticut Institute for Education, Training and Research was formed. It has shared the hospice philosophy and the skills and experiences of the staff through a variety of educational techniques. Seminars and courses have been offered on clinical and administrative matters. Videotaped training programs for hospice staff have been made available, and publications have been prepared to clarify administrative and caregiving directions for local adaptation. By far the most noted educational offering was the film *As Long as There is Life,* which was issued in early 1980.

As the decade of the nineties dawns, attention is shifting toward on-site and hands-on training for professionals. Seven physician fellows receive training each year in conjunction with the Yale University School of Medicine. In 1989, 24 nurses were privileged to become Citicorp Nursing Fellows, each spending a week in classroom and hands-on instruction in both inpatient and home care. A large number of registered nurses in both inpatient and home care settings participated as clinical preceptors.

The Value of Volunteers. On August 16, 1990, President George Bush designated the volunteers of the Connecticut Hospice as the 223 Point of Light in his quest for 1,000 Points of Light marking personal service on behalf of others.

Connecticut Hospice volunteer manager Barbara Larson reported that the Connecticut Hospice, Inc., recognizes the value of utilizing volunteer staff in its efforts to meet its goal to provide quality care for patients and families. Caregiving and other volunteers supplement and support the paid staff.

"To do something meaningful" is the overwhelming reason for volunteering at the Connecticut Hospice, as 375 volunteers derive meaning, energy, and joy from working directly with patients and families or indirectly supporting them in many other roles. Volunteers come from varied sources, chiefly via word of mouth referral, to work in such areas as home care, inpatient care, pastoral care, the arts, bereavement counseling, the Cottage, and staff support for the hospice and the institute.

Volunteer Training. Direct-patient-care volunteers are given 16 hours of comprehensive training to help them to interact with a dying patient and his or her family in the broad spectrum of hospice caregiving. The training, which explores the multiple facets of hospice care, consists of lectures by staff and other professionals, films, and panel discussions with group participation. The patient-care volunteer may then choose to work in three main areas of direct patient care: the inpatient facility, the home care program, and the Cottage for the homeless (Larson, 1990).

Volunteer Bereavement Program. The Connecticut Hospice Bereavement program is run entirely by volunteers who follow up high-risk families by telephone and/or in person to assess their bereavement needs. Bereavement volunteers assist with monthly support meetings for bereaved families and act as members of the team through regular attendance at team meetings. Rahm Das submits the following: "If you want to learn about life, work with the dying." (Larson, 1990).

Rekindling the Hospice Nurse. In 1980, a task force of direct nursing caregivers was developed to plan a burnout prevention program, the result being a yearly, two-day retreat known as Rekindling Days. The retreat was conceived more as a time to share and explore than as a chance to solve specific problems or develop specific professional skills. The format is open-ended, with no right or wrong answers; it is an educational process designed to develop understanding and promote personal and professional growth. The program is mandatory for all direct caregivers, charge nurses, and supervisors. It is held away from the hospice premises in groups of less than 40 people and facilitated by a skilled professional from outside the staff. It is expected that the retreat will be an ongoing component of the nursing support program (Bailey, Carney, Grodski, & Turnbull, 1987).

FINANCIAL COMPONENT

The option of hospice care throughout the United States has become available to patients and families largely as the result of coverage by third-party payers. The principal sources of third-party coverage are Medicare, Blue Cross, private insurance companies, and Medicaid.

Medicare. In 1982, Congress passed the Tax Equity and Fiscal Responsibility Act, which, for the first time, provided payment of hospice costs for Medicare recipients. Although the new hospice benefit contained a "sunset" provision calling for review of the Act in 1986, Congress voted to eliminate this provision, essentially extending the coverage indefinitely (Abbott, 1988).

Under Medicare, hospice is primarily a comprehensive, home care program designed to provide all the reasonable and necessary medical and support services, including pain control, for the management of a terminal disease. These services include physician care, nursing care, medical appliances and supplies (including outpatient drugs for symptom management and pain relief), home health aide and homemaker services, therapies, medical social services, and counseling. Short-term inpatient care is also covered by Medicare hospital insurance when a patient receives these services from a Medicare-certified hospice. There are no deductibles or copayments. Except for limited cost-sharing for outpatient drugs and inpatient respite care, Medicare pays the entire cost (Abbott, 1988). Medicare coverage is available through certified hospices. As of May 4, 1990, there were 806 Medicare-certified hospices in the United States (Hospice Forum, 1990).

The Connecticut Hospice, Inc., is Medicare certified, and approximately 75% of its patients are covered by Medicare. For many hospices, total costs of giving care have exceeded the amount they have been reimbursed by Medicare.

Blue Cross. The Blue Cross and Blue Shield Association has issued a recommended plan containing "contract language" and lists of exclusions and limitations for its member groups to use for their national benefit accounts. This document is useful in determining the details of the coverage offered to both national and individual state and local accounts. Hospice services for a terminally ill member with a life expectancy of 6 months or less must be provided according to a physician-prescribed treatment plan (Abbott, 1988).

Medicaid. Medicaid reimbursement for hospice services was approved by Congress on March 20, 1986, as part of a mammoth Budget Reconciliation Act. Under this provision, hospice care may be provided to a patient who is a resident of a skilled nursing facility or an intermediate-care facility (Abbott, 1988). Though Congress has included coverage of hospice patients under Medicaid, whether such coverage occurs has been left to the individual states. In 1990, Representative Leon Panetta and 31 cosponsors introduced an amendment to make such coverage mandatory.

Corporate Coverage of Hospice Care. Many patients are covered through major-medical or other health insurance coverage. As of January 1987, insurance coverage of hospice care is mandated in several states. The General Electric Company was the first major U.S. corporation to provide insurance coverage for its employees needing hospice care (Abbott, 1988).

In 1989, a Hospice Association of America survey of Fortune 200 companies showed that most offered such coverage for employees and retirees too young for Medicare. Such private insurance coverage is included in major-medical policies offered by companies to employees and their families. In 1989, the Hospice Association of America reported that 78 major U.S. insurance companies offered such policies to their corporate subscribers.

Foundations. The American Cancer Society, United Way, and service associations, such as the Rotary Club, often donate or grant monies to hospice.

Philanthropy Funding. The Connecticut Hospice, Inc., relies heavily on donations to help provide unreimbursed care to those without insurance, to provide counseling services to patients through the arts and pastoral care, and to maintain nursing and medical care at a needed level.

Private Self-Pay. About 1% of the Connecticut Hospice care is paid for by the patient and/or patient's family.

If a patient is not covered by insurance, hospices generally seek special funding to cover costs, and no one is turned away for lack of funds.

Open System of Care. The open system of care is difficult to interpret to cost-regulating agencies. Because the true cost of hospice care becomes the total cost during the final weeks of life in all settings, it also includes care for the family in bereavement. There is an element of tragedy in the competition between settings in which one can do the work at lowest cost, instead of which can do it best: "Issues are seen by bureaucratic agencies in economic terms; proposed care can be easily wrapped in the paper of cost containment to the detriment of its principles" (Wald, Foster, & Wald, 1980).

Many hospices have elected to provide care without benefit of Medicare reimbursement because of the ethical dilemmas imposed by the Medicare hospice regulations. Generally the structure of the Medicare hospice regulations rewards cost-cutting without reinforcing the provision of quality care. The major dilemma comes when financial considerations lead to the withholding of appropriate care. This yoke of regulations makes a mockery of the hospice philosophy (Sherman & Finn, 1987).

The Future of Physician Involvement. Recent events, such as the adoption of the diagnostic-related-groupings method of payment by Medicare and others, has set limits on length of hospital stays and, therefore, the number of visits for which physicians may charge. Physicians in several states have filed suit against group insurance providers, such as Blue Cross, for insufficient payment (Abbott, 1988).

Hospice care underscores the patient's and family's right to decide to discontinue treatment when it is unlikely to produce healing results, or when quality of life is more important than length of life. While this decision may limit the physician's potential income, it enhances the physician-patient relationship from the standpoint of humanitarian concern for the feelings of all involved (Abbott, 1988).

Financial Dependency on Volunteers. Volunteers are an integral part of virtually all hospice programs in the United States. In addition to their critical role in maintaining the spirit of hospice, volunteers make hospice much less expensive than hospital care for the terminal patient (Friedman, 1979). The Connecticut Hospice program includes 375 volunteers in more than 40 different categories of work. Noncaregiver work includes reception duties, public speaking, and mailing, while caregiver work includes home visits, transportation for patients, counseling, and clinical duties.

EVALUATION

Periodic accreditation reviews by the Joint Commission on Accreditation of Healthcare Organizations (JCAHO) have served as a national, voluntary evaluative mechanism for the growing hospice movement. The Connecticut Hospice, licensed as a "Short Term Hospital, Special, Hospice" under the Connecticut Public Health Code, was the first hospice inpatient program to be accredited by JCAHO as a hospital. When standards were developed for hospice accreditation, Connecticut Hospice participated with other hospices in suggesting criteria, and it subsequently became accredited as a hospice.

Unfortunately, JCAHO decided in 1990 to give up its hospice accreditation program, thus creating a void. JCAHO accreditation is invaluable to insurance companies as they process hospice claims. How that void will be filled, if at all, remains to be seen.

Though governmental review programs do involve the meeting of certain criteria in order to secure and retain certification, this process does not really fulfill the same need for evaluation that JCAHO had filled.

Conclusion. In the final analysis, however, nothing surpasses the evaluation offered by patient family members who have found hospice service helpful in meeting their needs at a most difficult time in their lives. Hospices find that from the moment of entry into hospice care to bereavement, both the patient and his or her family appreciate the warmth, listening, and care for the family that is provided. Hospice care provides an opportunity for genuine self-fulfillment during the final stretch of the journey through life. To maintain such appreciation is an important challenge for hospice people throughout the country.

REPLICATION

National Replication. The Connecticut Hospice, Inc., has served as a model for hospice organizations across the nation. The Rev. Edward F. Dobihal, Jr., formerly of the Department of Religious Ministries of the Yale-New Haven Hospital, notes that the success of Connecticut Hospice requires a sense of vision, coupled with the recognition that such a program is not a panacea or utopia. It requires a careful balance of the science of medicine and the art of care, and an understanding of the tensions that exist between them. There is a recognition that the world will not be made perfect for those who are dying or those continuing to live, but hospice will be a place where some patients and families can receive the best of care, where lessons can be learned, and where improvements can be made that can be shared with others who are serving the terminally ill in other health care systems (Dobihal, 1974).

RESOURCES AND REFERENCES

Abbott, J. (1978). Hospice: New way to help the dying. *A.D., 78*, 19-23.

Abbott, J. (1988). *Hospice resource manual for local churches.* New York: Pilgrim Press.

Bailey, B., Carney, M., Grodski, P., & Turnbull, M. (1987, July/August). Holding onto ideals in the face of reality: Rekindling the hospice nurse. *The American Journal of Hospice Care,* 31-35.

Bailey, S. (1987, November/December). The arts as an avenue to the spirit. *New Catholic World,* 264-268.

Craven, J., & Wald, F. S. (1975). Hospice care for dying patients. *American Journal of Nursing, 75* (10), 1816-1822.

Dobihal, E. F. (1974). Talk or terminal care? *Connecticut Medicine, 38* (7), 364-367.

Fisher, L. (1989). The home care people. The Connecticut Hospice Newsletter, 13 (1), 1-2.

Friedman, E. (1979). To make the road less lonely: The volunteer in hospice care. *The Volunteer Leader, 20.*

Hospice Association of America. (1990). *Hospice Forum, 5* (9), 8.

Larson, B. (1990). Philosophy Statement. The Connecticut Hospice, Inc.

Sherman, L. M., & Finn, W. E. (1987, July). Ethical dilemmas imposed by the Medicare hospice regulations. *New York State Journal of Medicine,* 379-380.

Wald, F. S., Foster, Z., & Wald, H. J. (1980). The hospice movement as a health care reform. *Nursing Outlook, 28* (3), 173-178.

Yoder, C. S., & Primer, M. H. (1989, January). A new dimension of hospice care: The Connecticut Hospice Cottage. *Caring,* 49-53.

For further information, contact:

The Connecticut Hospice, Inc.
61 Burban Drive
Branford, CT 06405
(203) 481-6231

12

Generations Assisted Living Homes: Miller-Dwan Medical Center
Duluth, Minnesota

with THOMAS M. PATTEN

The Generations Assisted Living Homes model of long-term care specializes in offering assisted living in houses for persons with Alzheimer's disease and related conditions. These homes are licensed Adult Foster Care and are structured to access funding for low-income (Medicaid-eligible) individuals.

DESCRIPTION OF GENERATIONS

Minnesota licenses two types of foster care: family foster care and corporate foster care. The Generations program is offered under the corporate license when the home is staffed by trained personnel working 8-hour shifts. The home becomes the home of the people who reside therein, and services are provided by outside agencies. Rather than being considered a mini-institution, where staff work and individuals are admitted, the Generations Assisted Living Homes are the home of the individual who lives there, and caregivers come into their home to provide services.

The Generations Assisted Living Homes are viewed as an alternative to institutional placement for persons who choose this alternative and meet the following intake criteria:

1. are diagnosed with an irreversible dementia;
2. do not need ongoing skilled nursing care (i.e., are medically stable); and
3. are ambulatory and unable to live independently.

The Minnesota Association of Homes for the Aging presented the 1989 Innovation of the Year Award for Community-Based Programs to Generations, located in Duluth, Minnesota. The program of the Miller-Dwan Medical Center is currently operating six homes with four residents per home. Two more homes are scheduled to open by 1991 in the Duluth area, each serving eight residents.

Although this model is currently specializing in the care of persons with Alzheimer's disease and related conditions, the model is not limited to this service. In fact, plans are underway to expand into services for the mentally ill elderly, ventilator-dependent housing, and head-injury-assisted living services (see Figure 12.1).

PHILOSOPHY OF GENERATIONS

The concept behind the Alzheimer's assisted living homes is the belief that although the underlying disease process of Alzheimer's cannot be treated, the symptoms associated with the disease can be effectively managed. Not unlike persons living with other chronic conditions, the effective management and treatment of the symptoms will result in improved quality of life for its victims.

The primary symptom of this disease is the initial loss of memory; gradually, victims are unable to adjust to environmental changes and eventually become incapable of meeting even their most basic needs. By providing a therapeutic program that recognizes the special needs of this population, persons are able to live their lives to the fullest, minimizing the impact of the disease process.

The Generations Assisted Living Model is built on the conviction that older persons, even those with extensive medical needs, can be served in the community setting. The least restrictive and most homelike environment possible influences positively the quality of life and will to maintain maximum independence. Institutional settings have been overutilized and continue to be so because there are no other alternatives for persons of moderate and low incomes.

**ASSISTED LIVING MODEL
THE GENERATIONS PROGRAM
MILLER-DWAN MEDICAL CENTER
DULUTH, MINNESOTA**

OLDER PERSON ASSESSED, AND DETERMINED IN NEED OF
SUPERVISION, ASSISTANCE AND PERSONAL CARE TO REMAIN IN THE
COMMUNITY

THE INTEGRATED CARE PLAN

THE KEY IN COORDINATING THE SERVICES PROVIDED IN A MANNER THAT BRINGS
MAXIMUM BENEFIT TO THE RESIDENT AND EFFECTIVELY INTEGRATES THE TEAM OF
PERSONS PROVIDING SUPPORT AND ASSISTANCE

CARE GIVING TEAM

ADULT FOSTER CARE WORKER PROVIDES:

- FOOD
- LODGING
- PROTECTION
- SUPERVISION
- HOUSEHOLD SERVICES

AND CAN PROVIDE

- PERSONAL CARE
- HOUSEHOLD/LIVING SKILLS
- MEDICATION ASSISTANCE
- ASSISTANCE SAFEGUARDING CASH RESOURCES

PERSONAL CARE ASSISTANT PROVIDES:

- BOWEL & BLADDER CARE
- SKIN CARE
- BATHING,GROOMING,ETC.
- RANGE OF MOTION EXERCISE
- RESPIRATORY ASSISTANCE
- TRANSFERS
- TURNING/POSITIONING
- CLEANING EQUIPMENT
- DRESSING/UNDRESSING
- ASSISTANCE WITH FOOD, DIET, NUTRITION
- ACCOMPANYING PERSON FOR MEDICAL
  TREATMENT,ETC.
- OTHER DAILY LIVING NEEDS

FUNDING FOR SERVICES

ADULT FOSTER CARE: MINNESOTA SUPPLEMENTAL
ASSISTANCE (MSA) AND PRIVATE PAYMENT

MSA AVAILABLE FOR INCOME ELIGIBLE OLDER PERSONS,
BASED ON DIFFICULTY OF CARE ASSESSMENT WITH STATE
MAXIMUM RATES ESTABLISHED

PRIVATE PAYMENT RATE SET AS DESIRED BY FACILITY

MEDICAL ASSISTANCE:

AVAILABLE FOR PERSONS WHO QUALIFY; PERSONAL CARE
SERVICES DELIVERED BASED ON A CARE PLAN AND INCLUDE
DOCTOR'S ORDERS; BASIC THRESHOLD ESTABLISHED BY
STATE, WITH A HEALTH CARE COST ASSESSMENT USED IF
ADDITIONAL FUNDS ARE NEEDED TO PROVIDE CARE

Figure 12.1. Assisted Living Model, The Generations Program, Miller-Dwan
Medical Center. Used with permission.

THE HISTORY OF GENERATIONS

The award-winning program began in 1981 when newlyweds Thomas Patten and Joyce Hidahl moved to Twig, Minnesota, to start a new life-style based on low-consumption living and the desire to provide a group home for the elderly. Prior to this, Tom worked as a county social worker and was the family caregiver for his grandmother. Joyce, an occupational therapist, worked at a local rehabilitation facility and was also the family caregiver for her grandmother. Their similar past personal and professional experiences led them to offer services for the elderly in their own home, called Twig House.

Their first resident was referred with a diagnosis of Alzheimer's disease and was "dishonorably" discharged from a nursing home for aberrant behavior. Soon Twig House became known as "the place" for the elderly who did not "fit" into the traditional nursing home program because their needs required a social, behavioral, and environmental approach rather than a more traditional medical model.

In 1985, Miller-Dwan Medical Center, a multispecialty, city-owned, not-for-profit hospital, visited Twig House. The Medical Center's future projection was to creatively meet the needs of the increasing elderly population in nontraditional ways and outside hospital walls. Mr. Patten was asked to join the staff to create community responses for the growing need for community-based long-term chronic care.

Thus the Generations Alzheimer's Residential Care Program developed out of need. According to the National Institute on Aging (NIA), as many as 4 million people are likely suffering from Alzheimer's disease. The NIA projects that with the steady growth of the over-65 population and the expected quadrupling of the over-85 age group, an alarming 14 million persons will be victims of Alzheimer's by the year 2050. These numbers indicate that Alzheimer's disease may be the biggest public health dilemma the United States has ever encountered. With the slow progression of Alzheimer's, many families are left destitute.

Miller-Dwan Medical Center has a strong commitment to offer care based on need, not ability to pay. Therefore, it is necessary to design services to permit access by low-income, Medicaid-eligible, persons. Generations services are so organized, thereby offering continuity of care even after a resident exhausts his or her personal savings.

A significant deterrent to utilization of community resources for older persons was the difficulty in accessing and managing a suitable payment system for those individuals requiring a continuously supervised setting but who could not afford to pay privately for services. The Generations Assisted Living Model demonstrates that care in the community can be delivered for the same cost or less than similar institutional care; it presents the argument that if a more desirable quality of life can be provided for older persons that does not exceed the cost of institutional care, there should be no conflict between the traditional public policy regarding institutionalization and noninstitutional care.

Compensating Environment. One of the keys to fulfilling the program philosophy of care is the development of a compensating environment for the persons who live in assisted living homes. A compensating environment is an environment that compensates for a person's mental and physical impairments and deterioration. Rather than being an obstacle to the continued independence of the person, the environment helps to compensate for limitations.

Based on work with an architectural firm, D. E. Stanius and Associates, Inc., and program staff of the Generations Assisted Living Homes, the following design considerations for the development of a compensating environment were applied to the Alzheimer's assisted living homes:

1. Design the home environment. The facility is designed with familiar architectural images commonly found in the neighborhood in which the building is situated. The interior is designed to seem as normal as possible to patients. Materials and finishes common in residential design are utilized to help residents feel like they are in their own homes.

2. Design entire facility on one level. A one-level facility provides accessibility to all functions to people in wheelchairs or with other physical disabilities.

3. Design space for private family visitation, including a guest bathroom. The families have a desire for private visitation away from other residents. There is also need for family/guest bathrooms. There is a possibility that the guest visitation space could serve a dual purpose by incorporating some of the experience centers (a special area, such as an office environment or tinkering bench) into this space.

4. Design private bedroom for each resident. Privacy is a high priority for family members and provides the resident with space that belongs to him/her. Staff recommends that bedrooms be small to encourage residents to spend time outside the bedroom.

5. Design for personalization of space. This includes designing a home environment that allows residents to bring some of their own furniture for their bedroom, possibly their favorite chair into the living room, and allowing them to provide their own memorabilia, photos, or favorite trophy to display in the living areas. An effort is made to preserve the dignity and self-esteem of residents. For example, a compartmentalized bathroom facility enhances privacy and self-esteem, and individualized brightly colored boxes on doorways to each bedroom can be used for mail and messages. Residents are even allowed to choose their bedroom color before moving in.

6. Design the kitchen/laundry experience center as "heart of the home" concept. The kitchen and laundry area are combined into one work area and Experience Center for the residents and are located in such a manner that there is visual control over all living spaces. Thus staff can work at this location and still maintain visual control over the residents. For example, a low counter built into the kitchen work area allows residents to sit in a stable chair and help with food preparation while sitting opposite the staff person. A table is provided near the laundry area so residents can help fold clothes.

7. Design experience centers into the home. Examples of Experience Centers are a tinkering bench, a place to work on automobiles, or an office environment. The compensating environment finds ways to engage residents in normal activities of daily living.

8. Design to meet emotional needs: Concepts include a front porch for sitting, incandescent lights in the bathroom for mood, attention to day lighting concepts, and understanding views and vistas on the site and capitalizing on them in the design; orientation of sitting rooms within the house to activity areas outside; use of color for depression avoidance; creation of a wandering path; and a deck, patio or three-seasons porch.

9. Design for security. The design includes electronic state-of-the-art motion detectors in bathrooms, electronic push-button lock release buttons for exterior doors and gateways, a push button in the bathroom, and electronic emergency call buttons from the bathroom and bedroom to staff areas.

10. Design for physical limitations of residents. The design includes rounded corners on all hard edges; smooth textures on walls; allowances for mobility to prevent tripping; a salon sink so residents' hair can be shampooed from a chair position rather than having residents bend forward; lever hardware handles on all knobs, faucets and door handles; cabinets and shelving positioned to avoid high or extremely low reaches; handrail safety bars in the bathroom, tub room, corridor, and other locations; and radiant heat in bathrooms to warm surfaces of all fixtures.

11. Design for hearing impairment. Isolate all furnace and air-handling systems as much as possible since they create a high background noise. Provide sound-absorbing finishes, such as carpeting and acoustic material on the ceiling, to deaden sound. Orient rooms that may have open windows away from high automobile-traffic areas.

12. Design for visual impairment. Provide generally higher levels of lighting and glare-free surfaces. Provide task lighting under cabinets in kitchen and bathroom; well-lit bathroom mirrors; and well-lit entryway, garage, and exterior areas. Incorporate a large clock and calendar in the living space.

13. Design for high- and low-functioning residents. The facility accommodates both high- and low-functioning residents so the design, of course, must accommodate both types. The Experience Centers, television, and wandering path are extended for high-functioning residents. The low-functioning residents will require less activity, but need other design features, such as those to accommodate incontinence problems. This is done by providing a cleanable carpet that could be easily removed (i.e., is not glued down) and a water-resistant subflooring so stains and odors cannot penetrate the flooring beneath the carpeting. Toilets could be readily accessible from public areas, as in a guest bathroom.

14. Design for handicapped accessibility throughout.

15. Design for concept of visual clues. Changes in carpeting color can be used to identify specific paths people may want to follow (i.e., to the bathroom) or to indicate areas that are off limits. The wall and floor contrast visually to prevent any visual confusion. Bathroom doors may be cued in a bright color or accent so residents can easily identify them, and memorabilia may be put near the resident's bedroom door for ease of identification. Toilet seats may be painted red as a visual cue.

16. Design for staff needs. This process includes installing electric and gas meters at the exterior of the home so as to prevent interruptions during the day; an electronic surveillance system or electric lock system; the use of portable telephones; a central vacuum cleaning system; redesigned toilet-flush valve system so that it is tamper resistant; an office desk work area in the kitchen; and deluge hot water fill in the bathtub.

17. Design for safety. The kitchen has a cabinet for all appliances and a lockable medicine cabinet. Individual hand-held shower heads and grab bars are in bathtubs and showers. All thermostats are tamper-proof. All appliances, refrigerator, stove, and freezer are lockable. Tamperproof caps are on all electrical outlets, night lights, emergency light packs in case of power failure, and front-facing controls on gas or electrical ranges. Electrical outlets are located at the floor line so that it is difficult for residents to bend over and reach them. Exterior hand rails are on any sloped sidewalks or pathways on each site.

ARRAY OF SERVICES

The Generations model maintains the older person in the most independent housing setting possible—individual homes—and organizes and delivers the health and social services in that setting. Thus the older person does not need to "progress" to more restrictive health care settings as frailty increases.

Generations provides a home setting with familiar furnishing and routines that are comforting to people with memory and orientation problems. The home is specifically designed to enable residents to function normally. The program provides 24-hour supervision and household safeguards for security, yet residents have the dignity and freedom to pursue their usual activities. These normal daily activities reinforce who they are and help maintain their sense of self. For example, if a person is used to staying up at night, falling asleep watching television, and sleeping in the next day, this routine is continued. Having only eight residents per home permits such flexibility. The Generations model structures the day to encourage residents to continue their usual life-style routines.

Family members are involved in the planning and ongoing review of their relative's care and have formed a program called GIFT (Generations Involving Families Together). GIFT meets on a regular basis, and families take turns providing weekly programs for residents. They have held fund-raisers to purchase a van to transport residents to community activities. Family relationship is respected and supported by a professional team composed of the medical director, psychiatric consultant, registered nurse, social worker, and occupational therapist. All caregivers are trained and certified home health aides.

Specific advantages of the Generations model are:

1. It is reimbursable for low-income individuals.
2. It utilizes existing community housing, and no special building or zoning requirements are needed, facilitating ease of startup. The small number makes it a reasonable proposition in either a rural or urban area without a costly market analysis.
3. The model is not disease specific and can serve a variety of populations needing assisted living.
4. There is opportunity for service excellence, a primary advantage. The service licensing, Adult Foster Care and Personal Care Assistance

programs permit the operator that rare opportunity today to act on all those thoughts about what could be done if only it wasn't for all those restrictive regulations. Direct care staff are challenged and invigorated by the opportunity.

The program components are designed to create a therapeutic environment that enables Alzheimer's patients to live satisfying lives regardless of the stage of disease progression. The following are the key program components:

- specially trained staff knowledgeable about the disease process, caring and compassionate in relationships with residents, and therapeutic in their approach;
- compensating environment, both social and physical, wherein residents can function optimally in meeting their own needs and continue their usual life-style activities; and
- holistic program of care that recognizes that residents come to the program to live, not merely to exist as persons who receive care.

The challenge in programming is not to "over-program" or "under-program." Doing too much may result in having the residents lose current skills and thus hasten the disease process. This approach may also teach residents to be helpless and dependent. On the other hand, too little programming may also result in loss of skills, both physical and emotional (boredom and depression), due to disuse if residents are not able to initiate activities on their own. Balance is the choice approach.

The unique experience of the Generations Assisted Living Homes provides staff and residents the chance to form caring relationships. With only eight residents per site, individualized attention and caring relationships are easily accomplished. The nature of the program is not to treat illness, but to care for and about people. Residents are encouraged to live each day to the fullest, not as patients, but as individuals with unique needs, while sharing a common need for relationships with people who accept them as they are.

By offering a program dedicated exclusively to a special needs population, Alzheimer's or other special needs group, it is possible to provide a quality of life that has not been heretofore available.

In Minnesota, corporate Adult Foster Care licenses a sponsor to provide care for up to four residents. The Generations model expands on this requirement by offering services in duplex settings where both units are licensed for four residents, thereby gaining some small economy of scale.

All residents receive the following Adult Foster Care services: food, lodging, protection, supervision, and household services. In addition, private-pay residents receive the following optional services: personal care and household/living skills assistance or training, medication assistance, and assistance in safeguarding cash resources.

Low-income residents who qualify for Medicaid receive personal care services in place of the optional services mentioned above.

Adult Foster Care. The Generations Adult Foster Care model uses basic adult foster care services for persons who are medical-assistance eligible, and both basic care and optional adult foster care services for persons who pay privately for their care. Basic services provide food, lodging, protection, supervision, and household services to functionally impaired adults in a residence. Optional services include personal care, household/living skills assistance of training, medication assistance, and assistance in safeguarding cash resources.

Personal Care Services. Personal care services are provided to medical-assistance eligible residents only in lieu of optional adult foster care services in order to supplement the adult foster care services in the Generations Home. Services include a range of personal care, such as assistance in bathing and dressing, preparation of meals, and medication assistance.

In Minnesota, personal care assistants (PCA) who provide personal care through provider organizations under contract with the sister Medicaid program are exempt from the licensing for home care agencies in Minnesota, but they must meet standards as defined by the Medicaid Program's Administrative Rule. PCAs are supervised by a registered nurse who is responsible for the personal and health care services they deliver. This is appropriate and required by Minnesota regulations.

Integrated Care Plan. Each person residing in the Generations Assisted Living Homes has an integrated care plan that addresses both the foster care and personal care services. The integrated care plan is developed by the team of persons providing services to the resident. A care plan is required by both the Adult Foster Care program as well as for Personal Care services. Payment for services are determined based on the care plans that document the care and services needed by the resident.

FINANCIAL COMPONENT

Private Pay. Older persons capable of paying for their services are charged a flat monthly fee for basic and optional foster care services that include all of the needed services defined above. These dollar amounts are subject to change annually. Private long-term care insurance policies may pay all or a portion of the care provided in the homes, and persons with policies should pursue this as a potential source.

Minnesota Supplemental Assistance (MSA). Minnesota Supplemental Assistance is a public assistance program that supplements Social Security income for low-income "aged" persons, and may be used to pay for adult foster care in Minnesota. In order to qualify for Minnesota Supplemental Assistance, an older person has to be financially eligible. A person who is MSA-eligible is automatically eligible for Medicaid benefits and does not have to apply separately for that coverage.

Funding can be a flat rate or determined on a difficulty of care assessment, depending on the policies of the individual counties. St. Louis County, where the Generations program operates, uses a difficulty of care assessment to determine the individual level of need and, therefore, the individual rate of payment for eligible adults.

The maximum monthly rate established by Minnesota MSA is $827 through 1991; prior to that time the maximum was $919. In January 1991, the MSA program will be funded by the state of Minnesota as opposed to being paid for by state and federal funding. All assessments will be done through a statewide difficulty of care assessment, and payment will be determined by that assessment.

Medicaid. In Minnesota, the Medicaid program is called the Medical Assistance program. As one of the many optional programs available to states, Minnesota participates in the Personal Care Assistant (PCA) program, which provides home care services to Medical-Assistance-eligible recipients who would otherwise require care in a health care licensed facility. Adult Foster Care homes are considered the eligible recipient's "place of residence" and therefore eligible for these PCA services.

Payment for home care services, utilizing the Generations model, is based on the comparable cost of care in a nursing home. Minnesota reimburses nursing homes based on a case-mix formula by which, after an assessment, an individual is categorized into one of 11 categories, A through K, with an accompanying dollar reimbursement rate. The current rate for community care, based on 1990 figures, extends from $991 for case mix level A to $2,208 for level K. Rates are subject to change annually.

The PCA provider organization is responsible for having a home care cost assessment (HCCA) done if the cost of care exceeds $1,325 per month. The public health nurse from the county pre-admission screening team does the assessment, and the individual is assigned a "case-mix" score that is most appropriate for the person's diagnosis, condition, and plan of care. The total payment of medical assistance home care services after the HCCA must not exceed the total monthly statewide average rate for the case mix classification most appropriate to the resident.

A principal advantage of the development of this model is that funding is in place, through the programs defined above, to make this model an alternative for low-income Minnesota residents as well as those able to pay privately. In the past, licensure rules have favored institutional placement (e.g., the older person becomes eligible for medical assistance through nursing home placement). Licensure tends to direct public dollars. Currently, with the licenses described above, both Adult Foster Care and Personal Care services can draw state and federal dollars for the income-eligible older person.

Although neither competitive regarding price, nor appropriate for someone needing ongoing skilled nursing care, the Generations model offers prospective residents the dignity of choice when their needs are primarily personal care, supervision, and a compensating environment. For individuals diagnosed with Alzheimer's disease or related condition, these services are "just what the doctor ordered."

EVALUATION OF THE
GENERATIONS ASSISTED LIVING MODEL

The program conducts a rigid self-evaluation that involves peer review and consumer feedback questionnaires. Success is measured by the demand for services, regular family survey, and financial performance. The demand for service far exceeds the capacity to respond. The waiting list is much longer than one could reasonably expect a referral to wait. At any one time, 50 names are on the waiting list.

A January 1990 family survey question was directly related to program goals and objectives of the Generation's *Assisted Living Manual.* Ninety-five percent of the respondents rated services above average. The financial proforma also demonstrates that the program is self-sufficient based on program earnings.

REPLICATION OF THE
GENERATIONS ASSISTED LIVING MODEL

The model as presented in this chapter is directly applicable to St. Louis County and the state of Minnesota. However, to the extent that other states arrange and regulate their services similarly, the model can be of value elsewhere as well. For replication efforts, Generations has prepared the *Assisted Living Manual* as a road map for use by other sponsors in developing the program in their communities. Because of the scale of the project, providing services for small numbers of older persons, the model has wide applicability for both urban and rural settings. The chief limitation of a manual and written communication is the inability to adequately convey the "feeling" of a model of service. Any persons considering the development of this program are invited to visit the Generations program of Miller-Dwan Medical Center in Duluth to "see" a program in operation at one of the homes.

The Generations Program staff are available to assist anyone in the development of their program, bringing the advantages of the demonstration lessons that include getting the program organized, as well as the evolution in staff selection, training, and development. Various consulting packages are available through the Generations program.

The Generations model is being replicated in several sites across the nation. The program has four principal advantages:

1. Living in homes/ease and low cost start-up:
   - Residential homes require no special building or zoning.
   - Only eight residents live in a home; therefore, its scale makes it workable in both urban and rural areas.
   - Normal family homes help persons cope with their disabilities and build on their strengths.

2. Access to funding:
   - Access to federal and state funding makes the program available to people of all incomes.
3. Financially sound:
   - It is a proven financial strategy that is self-supporting.
4. Appealing to families:
   - The tremendous market appeal of Generations attracts inquiries from families of persons with Alzheimer's disease and other chronic conditions.

In the Generations Assisted Living Homes currently existing, the persons served are older persons with Alzheimer's who are experiencing various levels of disease progression. However, the model need not be limited to the elerly since the program has applicability to any group of adults needing adult foster care services and personal care services in order to remain in the community and avoid institutionalization. The model is intended to be a generic model and has wide applicability for both older and younger persons who are "at risk" of institutionalization. The model is service integrated, combining the services of adult foster care and personal care. The setting is small scale, eight residents per home, rather than limited to a somewhat typical larger apartment building setting. However, the model is applicable to an apartment setting and can be financially sound and self-sufficient based on program earnings.

Generations provides an easy-to-implement package that includes consulting assistance to assure that the program is customized to special community needs. The program also offers a continuing network to receive updated information. The package includes the following:

- licensing assistance
- forms and contracts
- billing procedures
- pro forma
- care planning processes
- promotional publications
- on-site training
- presentations for staff, families of potential residents, and board members

RESOURCES AND REFERENCES

Patten, T. M. (1990). *Assisted Living Manual.* Unpublished program manual.

For further information on the Generations Assisted Living model, contact:

Thomas M. Patten
Generations Program Director
Miller-Dwan Medical Center
502 East Second Street
Duluth, MN 55805
(218) 720-1234

13

Concepts in Community Living: Assisted Living Program
Portland, Oregon

with KEREN BROWN WILSON

Concepts in Community Living is a social model of care that successfully supports very frail individuals in residential settings. The new assisted living program to enhance long-term care for the elderly allows an individual to live in his or her own private apartment with kitchenette and private bathroom. A 24-hour professional staff is available to provide care and service on an as-needed basis. This built-in service allows impaired, frail people to continue living in a home-like environment.

PHILOSOPHY: MERGING HOUSING AND SERVICES

The primary goal of Concepts in Community Living is to demedicalize long-term care and vary the amount of care according to the individual's needs in the person's home environment.

Individuality. The most basic assumption underlying this social model of care is individuality. Participants in the program are treated as individuals since the model recognizes variability in individual capabilities, has the flexibility to organize services according to individual needs, is able to modify services over time in response to changing needs, and exhibits the willingness to respect and accommodate individual needs.

Independence. Independence is another valued element of Concepts in Assisted Living that allows the right of frail individuals to make decisions. The program's philosophy to facilitate opportunities for decision-making is based on the premise that fostering dependency is inhumane and tends to infantize adults with disabilities thereby treating them as objects rather than individuals. Services provided mechanistically also increase the cost of care.

Assisted living maintains five principles essential to quality long-term care:

1. Choice: the ability to make decisions about one's life and having those decisions respected. To offer choice requires the development of options from which to select, the ability to organize information in such ways that choices are identifiable, the willingness to redefine or reorganize institutional operational modes, and the capability to follow through when a choice is made.

2. Dignity: acknowledgment by others that regardless of the level of disability, one is capable of enrichment of both oneself and others. Dignity implies worthiness and having a positive self-image. The program engenders feelings of worthiness by recognizing in tangible ways the uniqueness of the individual, accepting and supporting actions related to the need for expression of the self, fostering interactions that encourage mutual respect and courtesy, and focusing on individual abilities while accepting disabilities.

3. Independence: the power to make decisions regarding one's own life.

4. Privacy: the ability to control access to personal space. This principle promotes opportunities to control what happens with and in one's private space and recognizes that privacy extends to part of the self, including time not meant to be shared.

5. Homelike Environment. This principle generates a sense of family, community, and belonging where one feels comfortable and secure. The program allows the patient to keep furnishings and personal belongings that are comfortable and comforting, opportunities to become emotionally attached to a place and the people associated with it; and the creation of a setting that invokes memories and feelings of being at home.

HISTORY OF DEVELOPMENT

Concepts in Community Living evolved from a search to find new ways of providing ongoing support for the frail elderly and severely physically disabled because of concerns regarding increasing demands for service, rising costs of service, increasing consumer dissatisfaction with the medical model of long-term care, and increasing emphasis on quality of life.

In 1982, Oregon elected to support a pilot project to explore the viability of a new type of specialized living for frail elderly: a humane, cost-effective alternative to the medical model of custodial care. At that time housing developers had little interest in building foster homes, but serendipity was at work. Events drew together a group of people who had decided to build some sort of senior housing, and a partnership was formed. However, it was quickly apparent that getting a certificate of need for nursing home beds was out of the question and that the market was too saturated to absorb another traditional congregate project. Clearly something else had to be done if the partnership were to proceed.

A New Option. The most obvious solution was to build something responsive to consumer need for services and preference for remaining "at home." By merging concepts related to consumer preference (to receive care at home) and need (consistent access to a wide range of services 24 hours a day), a new approach to specialized housing was envisioned. Clearly, the key in conceptualizing this model was in the merger of design and services to support frail individuals in a setting that promoted principles they highly valued: privacy, independence, choice, dignity, individuality, and a normal home-like environment.

This concept was idealistic and not very conventional for the times. For the next year, the partnership worked on a package for financial lenders. Conventional financing proved illusive. The planning team was relatively inexperienced, had limited personal resources, and was proposing a project that had not been tried before. At the same time as the team was trying to attract lenders, the state housing agency decided to fund congregate housing for the elderly. However, the agency was reluctant to consider permanent financing because of the variances of the proposed model. This set a series of events into motion that unwittingly influenced the development of assisted living as a long-term care option for Oregon.

Implementing Assisted Living Housing. The first of these events involved the design of the building. Because the lending agent was financing "congregate housing," the project was required to have features consistent with the housing finance agency's definitions for housing units. This meant self-contained apartments with private baths and kitchens, lockable doors and private mailboxes, more common space, carpeting, and residential furnishings, among other things. Although these are standard requirements in independent living or congregate care programs, in 1982 they were unheard of in licensed care facilities.

A second event was a partnership decision to request licensure by the state of Oregon. At that time congregate care was generally defined as an option for moderate- and upper-income persons who had made a life-style choice to purchase living arrangements that included shelter with all utilities paid, security, maintenance, meals, recreation, housekeeping, and linen and laundry services. The partners' analysis of trends in the industry, the state's policy to expand the array of alternatives to nursing home placement, and personal experience in meeting elderly relatives' care needs suggested a wider range of services was needed. This meant licensure.

The third event was the lack of experience of both the project developers and the financing agency. The concept of having a variable service package and an inclusive-tiered rate structure was based upon a desire to broaden the potential market for a "new product" and personal reluctance to nickel and dime consumers. Consumers, in cooperation with case managers, could anticipate, plan for, and periodically review plans for needed services.

At this time, absolutely no one in the state was paying much attention to the 100-plus-unit housing project. Most assumed it was just another congregate care facility that might never be filled. As construction proceeded, many issues emerged and conflict raged among bureaucratic entities in deciding what type of building it was to be and who could live in it.

Senior and Disabled Services Division staff was skeptical of the project's merit. Even though residential care rules did not prohibit the development of the project as it was envisioned, licensing staff were nonetheless apprehensive about many of the design features and, more importantly, the scope of services planned for residents.

Design features that promoted the most controversy were those perceived to make the project more appealing to frail individuals who really wanted to remain at home, namely lockable doors, kitchens, individual heat controls in the living units, and carpeting. The commonly expressed opinion of the licensing staff was that these features were neither needed nor safe for frail individuals. Only after months of heated exchange was an exception granted by the Senior and Disabled

Services Division for the presence of stoves in resident units. This proved to be a key turning point in state policy.

Breakthrough in State Policy. The licensing staff expressed concern that the services proposed for the new project would mean that the facility would function as an unlicensed nursing home. Although existing rules generally permitted provision of most types of personal care, there were other areas where assistance was more restricted. Specifically, these restrictions had to do with mobility, incontinence, assistance with eating, need for nursing care beyond a period of eight days, impaired judgment, and medication administration.

Careful interpretation of the rules suggested that the restrictions were not explicitly stated. In the final analysis, it appeared the capacity to provide any routine nursing care task could be read into the rules or handled through the intermittent use of home health services. Thus variability in the range and intensity of services was in fact possible if the existing residential care rules were very broadly interpreted.

UNDERLYING PRINCIPLES OF ASSISTED LIVING

A Place of One's Own. Creating small private apartments with kitchens, baths, and locking doors was only the first step in normalizing the environment to make a home. It was just as important to actively encourage residents to furnish their apartments with their own belongings, including towels and sheets. Having their own things increased the residents' emotional attachment to their personal space.

Common Space. The expansion of common space for the use of residents was deemed important. Furnishings throughout the building are the same as those found in any home. Adaptations were made to cue those needing assistance in finding their way, to respond to episodes of incontinence, and to support physical limitations of residents.

Tailoring Service to Individuals. The model changed the language of service provision. Patients became residents, beds became units, and care became services. Changing the language made it less daunting to envision support provided in a more humane, cost-effective way. By recognizing variability in individual capabilities and organizing services according to individual need, the opportunity existed to accommodate a wide range of needs over time.

One of the greatest criticisms of institutional care has been the lack of ability to respond to the individual. To avoid the routinization of care provision, the decision was made that the service needs of every resident would be assumed to be unique. A typical package of basic service might include meals, housekeeping, laundry, and intermittent personal care; however, service was perceived in terms of interchangeable units combined in different ways for different individuals. The overall effect is not to have a standard service package, but to maintain the capability to deliver basic services to all residents at all times. Practically speaking, being able to accommodate the changing needs of the residents requires a monthly evaluation of service needs, with adjustments in the level and cost of service made accordingly. In this way, the concept of aging in place can be implemented more successfully for a frail population.

Shared Responsibility. Independence is encouraged by expecting the residents to do as much for themselves as possible. Meeting needs is a shared responsibility designed to encourage residents to make decisions, including those entailing risk, to improve the quality of their lives. Shared responsibility also means greater potential liability. The key to this dilemma was to plan in terms of managed risk—that is, the goal of shared responsibility is to lay out options in such a way that residents or their families could understand the consequences of a decision. Doing so means that more time is spent exploring options, talking about them, and aggressively seeking an agreed level of risk for an individual resident. It requires knowledge of resident capabilities, proactive planning to support those abilities, and alertness to conditions that might alter the agreed-upon level of risk. This notion of managed risk has not increased liability insurance in Oregon between 1982 and 1989.

Empowerment. The goal of assisted living was to reorganize the delivery of services so that choices were available and identifiable. For example, regulation required the longest time to pass between meals in licensed facilities to be no more than 14 hours. Typically, for the sake of efficiency, dinner and breakfast times were set accordingly and residents were told when meals were available. Rather than tell residents that meals were available at fixed times, choice as to when a resident could eat was offered by serving meals during designated time periods three times a day. Organizational efficiency is relatively unaffected, and perhaps even improved, by spreading demand more evenly across serving periods; yet, the resident chooses when to eat during that time. Choice is available for virtually every area of service, thereby empowering each resident to take control as to what time he or she would receive a service. Giving the resident control over time and how and when services are received is a critical principle of assisted living. This is complimented by providing resident control over space as well.

In sum, assisted living housing responds to some fundamental American values. A strong cultural preference for privacy exists in the United States. Providing a defined private space over which the resident controls access is the most obvious way of acknowledging the need and right for privacy. Private rooms, shared only by choice, with lockable doors allows privacy. It is equally important to train staff members to respect that need by have them request permission to enter that space and not interfere with how that space is used.

New State Policy. The first assisted living project in Oregon operated for nearly three years as an option available only to those able to pay privately. Gradually, the range of services was expanded and the limits of the project's license were tested. Conflict continued with the licensing regarding the type of residents (level of impairment), intensity of services (nursing tasks), and environmental features (kitchens). At various times, the licensing agent enlisted the aid of other regulatory units to support a more narrow interpretation of the regulation. The licensing agent's position was challenged by other regulatory units and client advocates. Finally, the administrator of Oregon's Senior and Disabled Services Division determined that a broad interpretation of the rules was acceptable given the special capability of the project to meet the residents' needs.

ARRAY OF SERVICES

In order to demedicalize long-term care, a social model of care has been designed, with services varying in the level of support in accordance to the level of ability for each individual served. The social model is divided into two categories:

1. Environmental, which involves the home or setting in which care is given, and includes housekeeping and laundry, and

2. personal/functional support services related to activities of daily living, medication assistance, and personal hygiene. Routine nursing tasks, such as injections, dressing changes, health monitoring, diagnosis, and assessment of clinical symptoms, are also provided.

Typically, these services vary in level of support provided, depending on the individual's level of ability in a particular domain (ranging from minimally independent to totally independent). Many of the desired environmental and programmatic characteristics of assisted living may be summarized as including:

- a defined private, personally furnished living space with shower or bath and kitchen area
- lockable doors to living space
- interior and exterior that are handicapped accessible
- emergency communication system in each unit
- security system to protect from intruders and to ensure the safety of wanderers
- common shared space for dining and recreation
- defined external space for resident use
- attractive, noninstitutional furnishings in commonly shared space
- three meals daily, seven days a week (including special diets)
- laundry service
- opportunities for socialization
- medical transportation
- personal care to assist resident in performing all activities of daily living, including bathing, eating, dressing, personal hygiene, grooming, toileting, medication management, and ambulation, etc.
- routine nursing care and health monitoring
- behavior management services for residents who are resistive to care, physically or verbally aggressive, and who wander and have primary or secondary diagnoses of dementia with attendant functional or personality disorders
- ancillary services for medical care (physician, pharmacist, therapy, podiatry), banking, barber/beauty, social/recreational, and hospice.

Profile of Residents. After several years of experience in Oregon, a profile of the private-pay resident most likely to choose assisted living has emerged. The majority are at least 80 years old, with the average

age being 85. Many have significant physical health problems, such as Parkinson's disease, post-stroke paralysis, severe degenerative joint disease, insulin-controlled diabetes, or congestive heart failure. Other residents may be victims of dementia, including Alzheimer's disease. They may be mobility impaired or incontinent, need nighttime care, or lack the cognitive ability to live without 24-hour supervision.

The residents are generally not permanently bed-bound and do not need continuous skilled nursing care. While they may be verbally or physically aggressive, they are not unpredictably violent toward themselves or others. Many exhibit symptoms of behavioral or psychosocial problems that make social interaction difficult, yet they enjoy and benefit from social contact.

OREGON'S ASSISTED LIVING
SERVICE PROVISION RULES

The need for service by patients in assisted living homes may vary from basic support with activities of daily living to more intensive personal and nursing care. This variability in need is the basis for the range of service specified in the new assisted living rules in Oregon listed below, which have been adapted from *Administrative Rules for Residential Care Facilities/Assisted Living Facilities,* State of Oregon.

1. Capability of assessing, planning, implementing, recording, and evaluating for necessary support services of resident's choices and independence.
2. Capability of providing or coordinating three meals daily, seven days a week, including diets and evening snacks appropriate to resident's needs and choices.
3. Capability of providing or coordinating personal and linen laundry, including incontinent laundry.
4. Capability of providing or coordinating opportunities of individual and group socialization and to utilize community resources to normalize the environment for community interaction.
5. Capability of providing or coordinating medical and social transportation.
6. Capability of providing or coordinating personal care to assist the resident in performing all activities of daily living, including bathing, eating, dressing, personal hygiene, grooming, toileting, and ambulation.

7. Capability of providing or coordinating routine nursing care, such as medication management, injections, nail and skin care, dressing changes, health monitoring, nonskilled catheter care, and other nursing tasks as might be delegated under the (Oregon) Nursing Delegation Act.

8. Capability of providing or coordinating services for residents who have behavior problems requiring ongoing staff support, intervention, and supervision.

9. Capability of providing or coordinating the ancillary services of medically related care (e.g., physician, pharmacist, therapy, podiatry, banking, barber/beauty, social/recreational opportunities), hospice, and other services necessary to support the resident.

10. Capability of providing or coordinating the household services essential for health and comfort of residents (e.g., floor cleaning, dusting, and bed making).

FINANCIAL COMPONENT

Flexible Cost. Flexible cost is a vital attribute of assisted living and is determined by the level of care necessary for an individual to maintain independence. Whereas nursing home costs are based on a daily bed rate, assisted living costs are determined by the assistance one requires. As assistance increases or decreases, so does the cost. To date, assisted living costs have been about 20% less than traditional institutional care for both private- and public-pay clients. Some residents pay with private funds, while others are Medicaid clients. Assisted-living units are expected to replace about 40% of the current nursing home beds in Oregon.

Oregon is in full support of assisted living and is presently developing rules and regulations that will assist both existing programs and those interested in new projects. Five levels of payment, ranging from approximately a low of $800 to a high of $1600, have been established. The rate of payment is to be determined by client impairment level. Projections in Oregon based upon priority placement criteria indicate the average payment will be $1275. This includes a 5% quality incentive payment to be paid when agreed-upon client outcomes have been achieved. The intent of the incentive payment is to encourage providers to focus upon improving or maintaining functioning of residents, while recognizing the need to pay for the additional services required by more impaired individuals.

The quality incentive payment is only one of the unique features of the planned payment system. The provider will conduct a regular review and update of the service plan. Quarterly adjustments in the rate of payment for Title XIX residents will be made, if appropriate, based on the results of these interviews and service plan adjustments. Title XIX residents will have their needs reviewed independently at 6-month intervals by their case manager to determine if the rate of payment is appropriate. The goal is to facilitate payment changes, to more accurately reflect actual resident service needs.

EVALUATION

Demonstration Model. In the spring of 1987, Oregon's Senior and Disabled Services Division elected to support a Medicaid demonstration project as part of its community-based care waiver program. This decision was based on a proposal submitted to the division by the program director to provide assisted living for Medicaid clients. The goal of the project was to demonstrate the viability and efficacy of assisted living for Medicaid clients eligible for nursing home placement. Specifically, the state sought to place clients in specially designed congregate housing with intensive personal and nursing services. The Medicaid clients targeted for the program were those difficult to place and/or with significant behavioral problems.

Evaluation Conclusions. After an evaluation of the project, the state concluded that the clients placed in the assisted living project showed significant overlap in characteristics with nursing home patients. Both anecdotal and statistical analysis indicated improved client outcomes, particularly in mobility, orientation, use of restraints, and stability of placement. Cost to the state was approximately 80% of the area nursing home rate and 20% more than the average foster home rate. As a result of the demonstration, Oregon decided to actively pursue a policy of promoting the development of assisted living as an option for serving frail functionally impaired older persons.

REPLICATION

A major question in regard to assisted living project is what size seems to work best. In the classic sense, the size of a project is best determined by market demand. However, from a resident point of view, small projects may be more desirable in order to keep with the goal of having home-like units. Financially, depending upon local circumstances that might increase either operating or property costs, 20- to 25-resident projects seem to be about the smallest size of freestanding assisted living projects that are viable. Conversely, larger size projects may be able to provide a wide range of services. Projects larger than 100 units may present unique problems for client functioning and staffing efficiencies. For units attached to other projects (e.g., nursing homes or congregate care), it is less clear as to how many units are most desireable. It is clearly possible to mix congregate and assisted living services in a building or to include assisted living as one component of housing in a campus-type setting.

Cost of Construction. There are some general principles related to the cost of new construction and the rehabilitation of congregate and nursing homes. New development costs, including land, construction, fixtures, common area furnishings and equipment; systems development charges; permits; architectural fees; survey costs; financing; and pre-opening, marketing, and rental costs might be expected to range from $35,000 to $50,000 per studio unit for low- and moderate-income projects.

Cost of Rehabilitation. Rehabilitation costs vary, depending on the structural changes required. Congregate care projects are less expensive, generally requiring only some modification of baths and the expansion of common space to accommodate services. These basic costs might be expected to average around $2,000 to $10,000 per unit, depending on the changes required. In most instances, the cost of rehabilitating existing housing units can be recouped by the increased revenue from an assisted living project in the same period of time that is required to absorb cumulative losses in new construction.

Costs of Conversion. In contrast to rehabilitating existing housing units, nursing home conversions require more plumbing and electrical modifications. Generally, about 30 to 40% of the bed capacity is lost due to the larger private living and common space requirements. The average costs range from $8,000 to $12,000 per unit, but this range of costs is typically offset by reductions in operating costs of about 20%.

Oregon's Long-Term Plan for Assisted Living. Oregon is projecting the placement of 1,400 Title XIX clients in assisted living over the next decade. If assisted living attracts the same ratio of private to Medicaid residents as currently exists, some 11,000 additional units will be needed to meet the demand. While it is premature to determine whether these projections will be borne out, several hundred units currently are in the planning and construction phases. Between October 1989 and the closing months of 1990, three projects were licensed with a dozen in the process of licensing.

RESOURCES AND REFERENCES

Wilson, K. B. (1988a). Beyond loving care: Developing a social model of care. Portland: Oregon Gerontological Association.

Wilson, K. B. (1988b, Spring). Assisted living: State aims to fill gap in continuum of care. *Oregon's Journal on Aging,* 11.

Wilson, K. B. (1989, Spring). *The next bed elderly housing market.* Washington, DC: National Association of Home Builders.

Wilson, K. B. (1990). Assisted living: The merger of housing and long term care services. *Long-Term Care Advances, 1* (4), 1-7.

For further information on the Concepts in Community Living model, contact:

Dr. Keren Brown Wilson, President
Concepts in Community Living
5207 S. E. 80th
Portland, OR 97206
(503) 777-0907; FAX (503)-777-0978

14

The On Lok Senior Health Services Consolidated Model of Long-Term Care
San Francisco, California

On Lok Senior Health Services of San Francisco is a consolidated model of long-term care that has a history indicative of careful planning in dealing both with the constraints of resources and research and with the fragmentation of resources and services. On Lok has been created from the process of gradual implementation and a cooperative effort toward a shared vision. No other community-based program in the United States offers all supportive and medical (both acute and chronic) services through the same program, reimbursed by both Medicare and Medicaid capitated payments (Clark, personal communication, 1990).

PHILOSOPHY OF ON LOK

On Lok's goal is to maintain the frail elderly in their own community, preferably in their own homes, as long as it is medically, socially, and economically feasible to do so. The needs of the individual, rather than those of traditional reimbursement categories, determine the services that are provided. As a result, the model works to establish a flexible service system that allows direct service providers full control over all health and health-related services necessary to meet the needs of an exclusively frail population in the most cost-effective manner. Specifically, the program has three objectives:

1. to rehabilitate participants as much as possible through a variety of therapeutic services;

2. to maintain health and independence of participants by providing comprehensive medical, social, and nutritional services; and
3. to sustain the highest possible quality of life which controling health care costs through the flexible use of resources.

Seven model principles of the On Lok Senior Health Services program are as follows:

1. Participation is limited to frail individuals who meet functional eligibility requirements for institutional care.
2. Medical, restorative, social, and supportive services are integrated in a comprehensive service system designed to address the multiple, interrelated problems of the population.
3. All services are delivered in a manner that provides a coordinated response to meet the needs of the participant in the most efficient and effective way.
4. Service control is accomplished by a multidisciplinary team that assesses need and arranges for, or preferably, provides, all services required by the participants.
5. The service plan is designed to maintain each participant's residence in the community.
6. The administrative and service structure allows the program to adopt a risk-managed orientation to the changing needs of the participant.
7. Resources are integrated into a single fund, which is drawn upon to provide services. Reimbursement is no longer tied to its payer (Medicare or Medicaid) and consequently is not subject to the payment restrictions of either program.

ON LOK'S HISTORY OF DEVELOPMENT

Translated from the Chinese, On Lok means "peaceful, happy abode" and, for many, it also means contentment. Out of community concern, On Lok Senior Health Services began in 1971, to serve the frail, elderly residents of the Chinatown/North Beach/Polk Gulch neighborhoods in San Francisco with the nation's first adult day health care program.

During the late 1960s, a group of concerned citizens of this San Francisco area recognized the needs of the 18,000 elderly who had limited incomes and little or no command of the English language. Members of this aging group experienced physical impairment and confusion, even to the point of being unable to seek help, and lived in hotel rooms above nightclubs and behind stores.

The first solution considered, to build a nursing home, was quickly ruled out because of high costs for land and the realization that institutional rules and regulations would inhibit meeting the diverse needs of the multi-ethnic elderly population. The sociological determination that the services required for these different ethnic groups would encompass a large spectrum of options and should be accessible within the elderly's community led to the establishment of the day health center.

Gradual Implementation. On Lok began as a day health center for seniors in a renovated Broadway nightclub and has evolved into an all-inclusive, innovatively financed health care team with a multidisciplinary service team approach. During the first phase of implementation (1972 to 1975), the program was funded by the Administration on Aging as a research and demonstration project. In 1974, On Lok became a pilot project under Medicaid by a contractual agreement with the California Department of Health Services. This successful effort later led to the inclusion of day health services as a permanent benefit under Medi-Cal (California's Medicaid) once Medi-Cal designated the day health center as the core of On Lok's community care system. On Lok has expanded steadily, as shown in Figure 14.1, "On Lok's Health Program Development." A few of the project's milestones are listed below.

Expansion into a Continuum of Care. In 1975, On Lok's day health center expanded to two facilities and added in-home care, home-delivered meals, and housing assistance through an Administration on Aging Model Project grant. Upon becoming a legislated Medicaid program, On Lok (1978) received federal funding from the Office of Human Development Services to develop a program of complete medical care and social support for nursing-home-eligible elderly. The program expanded into the Polk Gulch area when the Bush Street Center opened.

Community Care Organization for Dependent Adults. In 1979, the Health Care Financing Administration authorized the reimbursement of On Lok with Medicare Section 222 waivers for the Community Care Organization for Dependent Adults (CCODA). In 1980, hospital and skilled nursing facilities services became part of CCODA thereby completing On Lok's health care package. The On Lok House was comprised of 54 apartments for the frail elderly, a third day care center, and a respite unit.

Risk-Based Community Care Organization for Dependent Adults. In 1983, On Lok became the first organization in the United States to

ON LOK'S Health Program Development

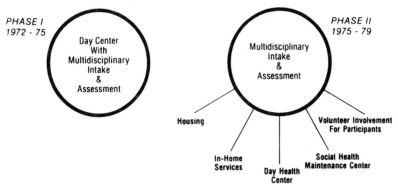

Community Care Organization For Dependent Adults

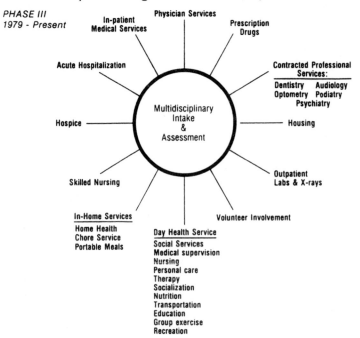

Figure 14.1. On Lok's Health Program Development. Used with permission.

assume full financial risk for the care of a frail elderly population. Program funding changed from cost-based reimbursement to fixed monthly premiums covering all services. On Lok diversified its funding sources to include Medicare, Medicaid, and private funds. The program was renamed Risk-Based CCODA to reflect the continuation of a complete service package and the change in program financing.

Beyond Demonstration Status. In 1986, landmark legislation gave On Lok approval to continue operating under its special Medicare and Medicaid provisions, conditional upon maintaining the program's cost and quality. On Lok thus became the first community-based long-term care program to move beyond demonstration status.

On Lok Replication Initiative. After 15 years as a "demonstration project," On Lok had the opportunity to prove that its unique model of service delivery and funding could work in other settings. In 1986, the Robert Wood Johnson Foundation awarded On Lok a grant for this purpose. The project enabled On Lok's staff to consult with other non-profit health care institutions around the country that were interested in adopting the principle underlying its funding model-provider assumption of financial risk in return for control over all services. These replication efforts will be discussed later in the chapter.

ON LOK'S ARRAY OF SERVICES

On Lok Senior Health Services of San Francisco is described as a consolidated model of long-term care in that it provides the complete continuum of long-term care services. The program's financing is also consolidated thereby allowing both maximum authority over and responsibility for client management. As a condition of participation, On Lok's clients are "locked in," meaning that enrollees must agree to obtain care solely from On Lok.

Multidisciplinary Team Work. A multidisciplinary intake and assessment team is the heart of On Lok's innovative program. Each day health center team is comprised of as many as 25 health care professionals and paraprofessionals who have extensive knowledge of each participant's condition. The team consists of physicians, nurses, social workers, rehabilitation and recreation therapists, nutritionists, and a paraprofessional staff. The team has complete control over services and may vary the setting in which they are delivered according to an individual's assessed need rather than by traditional reimbursement categories.

Thus, in delivering the program's services, the team uses case-management strategies intended both to minimize risk to the client's condition and to control agency costs. The team works together to assess each new participant's plans, delivers and continuously monitors care, formally reassesses all participants (at least every three months), and controls costs by tailoring care specifically to need.

Health Care Services. On Lok's services are targeted toward a high-risk, high-cost clientele: those elderly certified as sufficiently impaired to require nursing home care. Every service needed by a participant is provided by On Lok staff, ranging from friendly visits to intensive care and even surgery. If a client is hospitalized or enters a nursing home, On Lok staff continues to work with him or her. Nursing home stays may also include day health center attendance. On Lok staff provides:

- Primary medical care
- Skilled nursing care
- Physical, occupational, and recreational therapies
- Social services, including individual and family counseling, health education, and financial management
- Nutrition counseling
- Medical day care, including routine health monitoring and acute care
- Social day care (includes structured and nonstructured social activities)
- Post-discharge planning
- Transportation to and from centers and for other nonemergency services
- Meals, special diets as needed, and choice of Chinese or Western menu
- Personal care (includes showering, grooming, hair care, and laundry)
- In-home attendant and homemaker services
- In-home health care

Professionals under contract provide:

- Optometry
- Audiology
- Dentistry
- Psychiatry
- Podiatry
- Speech Therapy

Facilities under contract provide:

- Emergency medical transport
- Acute hospital care
- Skilled nursing care
- Laboratory testing
- X-rays
- Restorative and supportive appliances
- Medication

This lengthy list of services does not tell the entire story. Helping an elderly person live at home may also require delivering a prescription to someone's home, repairing a broken window, or calling a participant on the telephone for reassurance.

Supportive Housing. Although all participants are certified as needing nursing home placement, only 15% ever spend time in a nursing home. Housing is not technically part of On Lok's health-care package, though On Lok uses two types of supportive housing:

1. The On Lok House, which is a 54-unit facility that opened in 1980, provides accommodations for the community's low-income elderly. The house maintains a central dining area for those who are unable to prepare meals in their own kitchens. On Lok's Powell day health center occupies the ground floor of the building.
2. A second housing situation offered is "communal living," whereby groups of clients live together (with a companion) in privately rented apartments. All services are delivered by On Lok staff or provided under supervised contract.

Respite Units. On Lok also maintains two respite units in On Lok House. Participants living in the community may stay for a period of up to two weeks, thereby giving their families and caretakers a rest. The respite units are also utilized as transitional living quarters by participants who have been discharged from the hospital. The On Lok team continues to coordinate the care of clients requiring hospitalization or nursing-home placement.

The traditional long-term care system has frequently been criticized as too medically oriented and institutionally based. Research findings show On Lok's comprehensive program actually reduces hospital and nursing-home use. Since 1980, the average number of days an On Lok patient spent in the hospital has decreased from 9.9 to 3.3 days per year, a level comparable to that of the general population over the age of 65. The average admission rate, the number of admissions per participant per year, is only slightly higher than that of the general nursing home 65+ population.

Profile of Participants. On Lok serves the frail elderly—that is, those over 55 who are eligible for nursing home care. Clients, or "participants," must live in San Francisco's Chinatown-North Beach-Polk Gulch community, a 3-square-mile area.

Joining the On Lok program involves a three-part process: screening, assessment, and enrollment. First, the prospective participant and an On Lok social worker explore the program's features and eligibility requirements. Second, interested prospects who meet On Lok's frailty, age, and residency criteria receive a comprehensive health assessment. On Lok's multidisciplinary team thoroughly evaluates each prospective participant's physical, psychological, and social/environmental circumstances and recommends a treatment plan. Third, actual enrollment then takes place if the candidate agrees and if a nursing home level of care is needed, as confirmed by a representative from the California Department of Health Services. On Lok's participants are profiled as quite old, ethnically diverse, poor, living alone, frail, and functionally impaired.

Age. The average age is 80.9, with 42% between 80 and 89; 12%, 60 to 69; 31% 70 to 79; and 14% 90 and over.

Ethnicity. The participant population is ethnically diverse. About three fourths of the residents are Chinese, with the remainder being Filipino, Caucasian (many of Italian descent), and Black. About two fifths of the participants cannot speak English.

Income Level. The majority are poor, as assessed by the fact that 51% depend upon social security and 41% receive Supplemental Security Income (SSI). Only 10% have family support, 9% have investments, and 4% have pensions.

Living Arrangements. Over half of the participants are widowed, and two thirds do not live with their families. Sixty-four percent live alone, while 30% reside with a spouse or relative. Four percent live in a skilled nursing facility, and 2% reside with nonrelatives.

Frail and Functionally Impaired. Participants have an average of 5.4 serious medical diagnoses each. Three fourths are incontinent, and three fourths have extremity impairments. Most need help with bathing, grooming, dressing, and other activities of daily living.

ON LOK'S FINANCIAL COMPONENT

Integrated System. The On Lok model is also known as an integrated system since it integrates the financing, management, and provision of community-based care into one package. On Lok uses financial limitations to force prioritization of services in individual care plans. This is combined with case management that is consistent with the episodic clinical pattern of care associated with heavy users of services. On Lok bears 100% of the financial risk for the complete care of its enrolled participants.

Medicare/Medicaid. On Lok's primary financial resources include Medicare, Medicaid and the individual. Each of these sources pays a capitated or per-person monthly rate based on the individual's eligibility for Medicare and Medicaid. Participants who are fully eligible for Medicare and Medicaid pay nothing. Those who are eligible for partial Medicaid coverage (medically needy only) pay on a sliding scale. Individuals not eligible for Medicaid pay $1100 per month according to available 1986 data.

Under the special Medicare and Medicaid waivers, On Lok receives a fixed amount monthly for each participant in the program. These funds are managed by On Lok according to the service needs of the participant. The waivers also remove the usual restrictions on how Medicare/Medicaid funds may be spent. However, On Lok is responsible for the entire range of services in the consolidated model, including hospital and nursing home care, according to participant need. Once On Lok accepts a participant, he or she cannot be discharged by the program, although individuals may disenroll if they choose. Thereafter, upon enrollment, On Lok assumes responsibility for managing and paying for the full continuum of care needs for each participant.

The monthly capitation amount is paid by two of three sources. The amounts are computed in the following manner:

Medicare Capitation. The Medicare capitation payment of $790 per month per client is derived from the Area Average Per Capita Cost (AAPCC), which HCFA determines, multiplied by a "frailty adjustor." It is not subject to negotiation and is the equivalent of the average cost of Medicare-covered services for nursing home residents, adjusted for level of serverity.

Medicaid Capitation. The Medicaid capitation rate is a negotiated amount determined annually by the State Medicaid Agency and the program. In 1989, the Medicaid equivalent for Medicaid-covered long-term care services was $1,420. Cost data produced by the program and the state's experience with long-term care costs for a similar population are the basis for the annual rate determination.

Private Pay. Medicaid income eligibility is not a requirement for participation in the program. Private pay participants are charged the equivalent of the Medicaid capitation rate.

On Lok has remained financially solvent, even after assuming complete financial risk for all health and social services. In fiscal year 1989, monthly revenues from all sources averaged $2,210 per participant, slightly more than the cost of care. In return for this monthly reimbursement, On Lok provides all the needed health care for its clients—not only community-based long-term care and social services, but also primary medical care, medical specialty care, and even nursing home care and acute hospital care under contract. Hospital care is provided by several local hospitals for a negotiated all-inclusive rate between $799 and $800 per day (Beresford, 1989).

In view of the frailty of On Lok's participants and the need for coverage of catastrophic illnesses, On Lok must put its savings into a risk reserve pool. While On Lok has accrued savings, so have those paying the fees. The average payment from all sources was more than 12% lower than the estimated cost for this population in the traditional system (1984 Comparison Group Study, conducted by On Lok).

For the fiscal year 1985-1986, On Lok's total annual budget exceeded 6 million dollars. Direct services to the frail elderly accounted for 90% of On Lok's expenses. These expenditures covered day health services, inpatient care, in-home services, outpatient medical services, medical records and administration.

EVALUATION OF ON LOK

An extensive evaluation in 1988 by Zwadski and Eng revealed that On Lok services reduced hospital and nursing home use. The Kane and Kane (1987) investigation found that On Lok produced no mortality differences, but, instead, improved physical functioning outcomes, decreased nursing home use, and decreased acute-care days.

Reduced Hospitalizations. An earlier controlled study (Yordi and Waldman, 1985) viewed On Lok's performance for the period between 1979 and 1983 and found reduced risk of hospitalization (49% vs. 56%

over two years) and average number of study days in a hospital (2.1% vs. 2.7%). These findngs were attributed to the subacute care in On Lok's day health center. The study also reported reduced risk of nursing home entry (20% vs. 57% over two years) and study days in a nursing home (8% vs. 42%). Among those in community at baseline, reductions were also noted, with 14% vs. 26% entering a nursing home, and 5% vs. 13% of study days spent in a nursing home.

Fewer Nursing Home Admissions. Even for those living in nursing homes at baseline, reductions in study days spent therein were reported (42% vs. 86%). On Lok participants, in general, had fewer nursing-home admissions, and those admissions were of shorter duration. Variance in total public long-term care costs was reduced by about 40%. Adjusting for individual variance, On Lok clients costs were more that 20% lower. Acute hospital costs were reduced (24% of total vs. 39%), nursing home costs were reduced (11% vs. 42%), and community-based care was increased (65% of total vs. 19%). In other words, hospital costs were 51% lower; nursing home costs, 79% lower; and community-based care, 172% higher.

Other positive findings were a significant increase in homemaking skills, overall pattern of decrease in functional impairment, improvement as measured by psychosocial and physical Requirements of Living Indices, slight decrease in mortality, and increased use of out-patient and in-home services.

The above evaluation efforts conclusively agree that On Lok has been a consistently effective caregiving model from its inception to date. On Lok's costs have run between 8 and 19% lower than traditional care throughout the 1980s (Beresford, 1989).

REPLICATION OF ON LOK

Program of All-Inclusive Care for the Elderly: The On Lok replication initiative is called the Program of All-Inclusive Care for the Elderly (PACE). In December 1985, the Robert Wood Johnson Foundation awarded a grant to On Lok Senior Health Services for the purpose of supporting an effort to study the feasibility of extending On Lok's model of risk-based, long-term care services to the frail elderly in other parts of the country. This study marked the first step toward replication of the On Lok model in other settings.

The objectives of the feasibility study were:

1. to ascertain the level of interest in demonstrating a variant of the On Lok model;
2. to identify at least five organizations with the commitment and strengths to implement the model;
3. to secure service funding (waivers allowing Medicare and Medicaid capitated payments); and
4. to secure start-up funding for sites that seek to implement the model.

Site Interest. On Lok received over 180 letters of interest from hospitals, health maintenance organizations, state and local public agencies, long-term care facilities, and community organizations from across the United States.

Site Capability. Thirty-seven organizations completed the application requirements and requested full assessments. Nine sites were selected, and detailed site assessments were completed. Several of these sites are now in the implementation phase: Beth Abraham Hospital in the Bronx, New York; East Boston Neighborhood Health Center, Boston, Massachusetts; Providence Medical Center, Portland, Oregon; Richland Memorial Hospital/South Carolina Department of Health and Environmental Control, Columbia, South Carolina; Bienvivir Senior Health Services, El Paso, Texas; and Community Care Organization of Milwaukee County, Inc., Milwaukee, Wisconsin. In addition to Robert Wood Johnson Foundation funding, each of these sites was required to raise at least $300,000 in local matching funds. Of the four sites not eligible for Robert Wood Johnson Foundation funding, two have been designated: New Bethel Life, Chicago, Illinois; and Total Longterm Care, Denver, Colorado. Chicago and Denver obtained local funding for the development and implementation of the model. In addition, funding was secured to support technical assistance provided by On Lok/PACE. These two sites are operational in the fee-for-service phase.

Service Funding. On October 21, 1986, enabling legislation was signed under which Medicare and Medicaid waivers, like On Lok's, were granted to ten community-based public or nonprofit organizations for health services to be provided to frail elderly beneficiaries on a risk basis.

Start-Up Funding. In February 1987, On Lok embarked on the implementation phase. Unlike other multi-site demonstration initiatives, PACE has as its base an operating model: On Lok. To capitalize upon that advantage, On Lok is playing a large role in site start-up and project management. Three sites, East Boston Neighborhood Health Center, Beth Abraham Hospital, and Providence Medical Center, Portland, Oregon, secured start-up grants in November 1987. These sites have applied for HCFA waivers and will begin operating the model under capitation during 1990.

Each site must operate an adult day health center (ADHC) for 12 to 24 months on a fee-for-services basis before becoming eligible for waivers and capitated financing. Among the criteria for moving from fee-for-service to waiver financing are adequate development of the consolidated service model and enrollment of approximately 100 participants.

The replication projects have obtained grant funds to support development activities throughout the demonstration, to subsidize ADHC program operations during the early period when costs are high and census is low, and to pay for services that are not reimbursed under the traditional fee-for-service system prior to the waivers.

Replication of the On Lok Senior Health Services model is a technical and complex process. PACE has developed a framework for site development that consists of three transitional stages and nine development areas. The transitional stages provide a logical progression, with each stage building on prior service delivery, and administrative and financing experience. To progress through the stages, sites are required to meet PACE criteria in the nine development areas.

REFERENCES AND RESOURCES

Ansak, M. L. (1983). On Lok senior health services: A community care organization for dependent adults. *Pride Institute Journal of Long Term Home Health Care, 2* (1), 7-11.

Beresford, L. (1989, October 16). San Francisco's On Lok spawns similar programs across U.S. In *LTC Management*, p. 4. Washington, DC: Faulkner & Gray's Healthcare Information Center.

Kane, R. A., & Kane, R. L. (1987). *Long-term care: Principles, programs and policies.* New York: Springer.

Yordi, C., & Waldman, J. (1985). A consolidated model of long-term care: Service utilization and cost impacts. *The Gerontologist, 25* (4), 389-397.

Zwadski, R. T., & Eng, C. (1988). Case management in capitated long-term care. *Health Care Financing Review,* Annual Supplement, 75-81.

On Lok Brochures

Profile—On Lok Senior Health Services.

On Lok Senior Health Services (1978): The Risk-Based CCODA—A Financing Model for Long-Term Care, and Description of the Program.

PACE—Principles of the Model, and On Lok Senior Health Services.

For further information and On Lok brochures listed above, contact:

Program for All-Inclusive Care for the Elderly
1455 Bush Street
San Francisco, CA 94109
(415) 989-2578

15

Total Longterm Care
Denver, Colorado

with LINDA S. BARLEY

Total Longterm Care (TLC) provides health care services within an adult day health care center for those elderly individuals at risk of nursing home placement. A PACE program designed to replicate On Lok Health Services in San Francisco, TLC's mission is to promote the ability of the frail elderly to live in the community with dignity and independence. As an alternative to nursing home placement, TLC maintains participants in their own homes and provides support for family caregivers.

PHILOSOPHY: MAXIMIZING INDEPENDENCE
OF THE FRAIL ELDERLY

TLC provides comprehensive health care responsive to the needs of the individual participant. The program emphasizes helping the older person remain in the community, often in the same home he or she may have occupied and owned for many years. It is expected that by coordinating an extensive array of medical and nonmedical services, the needs of the participants will be met primarily in an outpatient environment, within an adult day health center, in their homes, and/or in an institutional setting. Such a delivery system will enhance the quality of life for the participants, and offer the potential to reduce and cap the costs of their medical care.

The seven guiding principles of the TLC Model are:

1. Participation is limited to frail individuals who meet functional eligibility requirements for institutional care.
2. Medical, restorative, and social and supportive services are integrated in a comprehensive service system designed to address the multiple, inter-related problems of the population.
3. All services are managed in a manner that provides a coordinated response to meet the needs of the participant in the most efficient and effective way.
4. Service control is accomplished by a multidisciplinary team that assesses need, and arranges for, or preferably provides, all services required by the participants.
5. The service plan is designed to maintain each participant's residence in the community.
6. The administrative and service structure allows the program to adopt a risk-management orientation to changing participant needs.
7. Resources are integrated into a single fund that is drawn upon in order to provide services. Reimbursement is no longer tied to its payer (Medicare or Medicaid) and consequently is not subject to the payment restriction of either program.

HISTORY OF DEVELOPMENT

A PACE program, Total Longterm Care was designed as a replication of the On Lok Senior Health Services in San Francisco. The On Lok program, which provides a comprehensive range of services, is characterized by a consolidated service delivery system, a multidisciplinary approach to managing each participant's care, and risk-based financing.

On Lok, described previously, has operated its model under 100% risk-based financing since 1983. In 1986, On Lok received federal and state congressional approval to continue operating under its special Medicare (Section 222) and Medicaid (Section 1115) waivers. In addition, the Health Care Financing Administration was authorized to award ten additional waivers to sites that met On Lok's criteria for replicating the risk-based model.

PACE Replication. The replication initiative, or Program of All-Inclusive Care for the Elderly (PACE), has, to date, selected eight of ten sites designated to participate in the demonstration. Total Longterm

Care, Inc., a nonprofit 501(c) 3 organization, participated in a site feasibility assessment in February 1988 and was designated to participate in PACE as the eighth site in August 1988.

Long-Term Care of the Elderly in Colorado. The demand for both acute and long-term health care services has been driven to a great extent by dramatic changes in the demographic composition of the population. Service needs tend to increase exponentially with age. Within age cohorts, service utilization is unevenly distributed, with functional impairment identifying those with greater need. The cohort with the highest service needs, those over 85 years old, is the fastest-growing segment of the population, having grown by about 50% between 1970 and 1980. Similar growth is projected for the next decade by the Colorado State Demographer for the Denver metropolitan area.

Nursing Home Alternative. The service setting most frequently associated with long-term care is the nursing home. Because Medicaid initially only paid for long-term care within the nursing home setting, the expansion of the capacity of that setting resulted. The increased availability of nursing home beds and the expected admissions of the frail elderly to those beds created the "spend down" phenomenon whereby those with savings spent their funds on long-term care until they became Medicaid eligible. During the same period, accessibility to long-term care insurance was minimal due to cost constraints and limited availability. These financial issues, combined with the stigma of being placed in a nursing home, served to create a new underclass of frail elderly individuals who impact Medicaid dollars.

Although nursing homes are categorized as health care facilities, their elderly residents may experience high rates of hospitalization. Improved service capacity would be likely to impact favorably on the hospital use rate of this population. However, the separate payer systems for acute care (Medicare) and long-term care (Medicaid/private) do not provide sufficient financial incentives for reforms in the service delivery in either arena. Rather than need, the service system is driven by reimbursement policy. With no coordination between payers, each simply seeks a means of containing its individual costs rather than pursue more efficient use of the total care funds available. Thus the needs of the frail elderly are not adequately met, and the cost to the Medicaid program continually increases due to increasing population, utilization, and costs.

Community-Based Alternative. Attempts to develop noninstitutional, community-based long-term care alternatives have met with limited success. Many efforts have been criticized for having neither the level of funding nor the level of coordination necessary to serve those with greatest need. Public policymakers must maintain the balance of resource allocation and cost control. Difficulties with "targeting" and the fear of "widening the net" are obstacles for policymakers, as evidenced by recent controversy over the Colorado Home- and Community-Based Services Program. Individuals seeking to use the options currently available in long-term care encounter a system that is fragmented, complex, competitive, and inaccessible.

PACE as an Alternative to Current Systems Within Colorado. Long-term care is an area in which innovation and experimentation are critical needs. Without substantive change, the already strained system will be unable to provide adequate care to the growing elderly population. No simple solutions are possible, but any response must include coordination of comprehensive services. This service package must be provided according to an individual's needs, and must promote greater independence and less reliance on institutional care. Total Longterm Care is an innovative program that meets these goals.

Currently in Colorado, the long-term care system is mainly supported by the nursing home industry and the establishment of the Home- and Community-Based Services Program. Additionally, the Home Care Allowance Program enables many elderly to remain within their own homes prior to the need for nursing home placement (see Table 15.1). While these programs serve the needs of specific elderly, there is room for an alternative to the current system.

Legislative Requirements. In order for Total Longterm Care to establish the PACE model in Denver, Colorado, the Colorado Department of Social Services must submit a Section 1115 waiver to the Health Care Financing Administration (HCFA). In January 1990, enabling legislation was introduced by Representative Wilma Webb and Senator Dennis Gallagher that would grant authority to the Colorado Department of Social Services to apply for these Medicaid waivers. That legislation, known as HB 1030, successfully passed through committees of both the House and the Senate and was signed into law by Governor Romer on April 16, 1990.

HB 1030 provided, for a 2-year period, a full-time equivalent position within the Department of Social Services to begin the process of

Table 15.1 Colorado Long-Term Care Service Element Comparison

Home Care Allowance (HCA) (Max. Cost $319/Mo.) (State financed)	Home & Community Based Services (HCBS) (Cost Avg. $600+/mo.) (State/Federal financed)	Total Longterm Care Service Model (TLC) (Capitation Est. $17000+/mo.) (State/Federal financed**)
Personal Care Services	Case Management	Multidisciplinary Assessment
Respite	Personal Care Services	Case Management
ADL Assistance	Nursing Home Respite	Day Health Services
	Alternative Care Facility	*social services
	Home Health Services	*medical supervision
	Electronic Monitoring	*nursing
	Home Modification	*personal care
	Transportation Hospice	*therapy (physical,
	(in home)	occupational, speech)
	Day Care	*socialization
	Homemaker Services	*nutrition
	Therapies (OT, PT, ST)	*transportation
		*education
		*group exercise
In addition to HCA and HCBS basic costs are:		*recreation
Hospital costs		In-Home Services
Medication costs		*transitional care
Physician costs		*post-hospital care
Nursing home costs		*preventive home health
Outpatient lab costs		*chore services
Contracted services costs		*portable meals
Podiatry		Palliative Care
Audiology		*acute hospitalization
Psychiatry		*inpatient medical service
		*physician services
		*prescription drugs
		*outpatient lab & X-ray
		*nursing home placement
		Contracted professional Services
		*dentistry
		*optometry
		*audiology
		**podiatry
		**psychiatry
Participants: 4,100±	Participants: 4,440±	Participants: approx. 300
Eligibility: Income/asset guidelines (no age limit); need	Eligibility: Medicaid income guidelines; over 18; LTC 101	Eligibility: Frailty screen, such as LTC 101; may be Medicaid or private pay

*These services may be required by an individual eligible for HCA or HCBS. The Department of Social Services incurs additional expenses through Medicaid if used. In the Consolidated Service model, the program is liable for these expenses; Medicaid pays only the negotiated monthly capitation for the participants.
**Additional capitation payment from Medicare (federal dollars) sets total monthly rate.

gathering the necessary information to write the application to HCFA for waivers, funding for the computer software changes to handle the capitated reimbursement system, and annual cost reporting. These provisions will continue as long as the program proves cost effective at the state level. If the project succeeds in proving cost-effectiveness for the state at the conclusion of the demonstration project, TLC will need to return to the Colorado General Assembly during the 1995 legislative session and submit by bill, a request permanent funding for the program from Medicaid.

Cooperative Negotiations. The passage of HB 1030 allowed the Colorado Department of Social Services to enter into cooperative negotiations with Total Longterm Care on the following three basic areas prior to submitting application for the 1115 Medicaid waiver to HCFA:

1. eligibility criteria of participant population;
2. capitation rate setting process for the waiver application; and
3. risk sharing during the three-year demonstration phase.

The Total Longterm Care date for submission of application for the necessary Medicare (222) and Medicaid (1115) waivers by TLC and the Colorado Department of Social Services was set for approximately November 1990. This date allows ample time for the Health Care Financing Administration Review Committee to process the waiver applications prior to the anticipated implementation date of July 1990.

PHASE I: STRATEGIC PLAN
TOWARD WAIVERED MODEL

Goals of Total Longterm Care during this fee-for-service phase (January 1990 through approximately July 1991) are:

1. to gain, as much as feasible, experience in cost-effective managed care of the frail elderly while serving the participants' needs through multidisciplinary team's case management. The PACE initiative by the Health Care Financing Administration includes monitoring of the replication sites by PACE in San Francisco. As part of On Lok's technical assistance to the Denver site, PACE will monitor, regularly, the utilization of all services for participants, as well as offer guidance and support as to how best transition the program into waiver; and

2. to successfully negotiate with the Colorado Department of Social Services and with HCFA an acceptable rate structure and a risk-sharing agreement to give Total Longterm Care time to refine service delivery and achieve efficiencies inherent in the consolidated service delivery model.

According to a detailed 5-year work plan, the initial phase of the project began the first day of operation through waiver implementation. It will take approximately 18 months for the project to go from the fee-for-service model to the waivered capitated model. The TLC center is newly built and is designed to serve approximately 120 enrolled frail elderly participants. Currently, the center is open Monday, Wednesday, and Thursday from 8:00 a.m. to 5:00 p.m. As soon as the census warrants, services will expand to five days a week, Monday through Friday. Eventually, after the second site opens, one of the adult day health centers will be open seven days a week to meet the needs of those requiring daily monitoring and/or care.

PHASE I: ARRAY OF SERVICES

During the fee-for-service phase, TLC provides the coordination of all health and health-related services needed by each participant. The multidisciplinary team of professionals and caregivers meets regularly to discuss any changes in the participant's needs and then coordinates the appropriate services. The Adult Day Health Center provides a wide variety of services not readily available at traditional adult day care programs. The following are included in the daily rate:

1. Personal Care. Services include bathing, grooming, hair and nail care, and toileting of those who need assistance.
2. Skilled Nursing. Services, provided by a registered nurse, include medication administration, catheter care, colostomy care, and nursing treatments and procedures.
3. Medications. In addition to the administration of medications to those needing assistance or who are unable to take medication by themselves, services include the coordination of all medications being taken with the primary, attending physician in order to decrease the possibility of poly-pharmacy.
4. Special Diets. Special diets (low-salt, soft, and pureed food), as well as diets designed for the diabetic and others, are available for the noon meal and two daily snacks.

5. Social Work. A masters-level social worker assists with the case management of all services on the participant care plan and assists the family and participants with applying for all federal and state programs as may be needed.

6. Recreational Activities. Led by a trained activity coordinator, these activities are geared to the particular levels of the participants and strive to stimulate and interest the participants in the world around them.

7. Other Services. Other services required by the family and the participant during fee-for-service are arranged and referred to outside certified agencies upon the order of the attending physician. These services are then billed directly to Medicare, Medicaid (if not covered by Medicare), or any other third-party insurer by the contracted agencies. The multidisciplinary team works very closely with the participant's attending physician and attempts to coordinate and control the allocation of these services in order to decrease a fragmented plan of care. In this way, the participant and family feel secure that the total health care and non-health care needs are being addressed by one agency.

These services are all coordinated by TLC and include:

- attending physician services
- physical, occupational, and speech therapies
- home health care
- lab and radiology
- medication ordering
- transportation to and from the adult day health center
- hospitalizations
- nursing home placements

PHASE I: FINANCING

Home- and Community-Based Service Program. During the fee-for-service phase, the program receives revenue under the Home Community-Based Service Program as a certified Adult Day Care Program. This certification requires that the agency meet specific regulations as dictated by the Colorado Department of Social Services. The Colorado Department of Health is responsible for the certification survey process, which is conducted annually by the State Department of Health, Health Facilities Division. This certification allows the program to have access to limited revenues.

During 1990 and 1991, the reimbursement rate from Medicaid for adult day care is $27.50 per day, or $13.75 per unit of 5 hours. All private pay participants are charged the same daily rate, and the program has made a policy decision not to shift any costs to the private sector.

The agency also is licensed by the Colorado Department of Health as a community clinic. Since the Adult Day Care model in Colorado does not allow for medication administration to participants, licensing as a community clinic was required in order for a registered nurse to administer medications to the participants at the Adult Day Health Center. The program does not bill Medicare, Medicaid, or any third-party insurers for the services of the community clinic as it was not cost-effective to obtain the proper certifications for only 18 months of fee-for-service operation.

The revenues realized from the reimbursement as an Adult Day Care program is not adequate to support the operations while the program transitions to waiver implementation. Therefore, it was necessary to research other funding options. The additional revenues needed for operation have been requested and awarded from local Colorado foundations. The dedication to improved quality of life for the elderly of Colorado by the Colorado Trust and the Presbyterian/St. Luke's Community Foundation is evidenced by the awarding of a total of over $1 million to Total Longterm Care over a 5-year period. During this time, the program will gain experience in managed care procedures in order to be as cost-effective as possible while providing the needed services under waiver.

Admissions Criteria. In order to qualify for Total Longterm Care, an individual must be eligible financially and functionally for long-term care as defined by the Colorado Department of Social Services if the payer is to be covered by Medicaid under the Home and Community-Based Services Program, Adult Day Care. Any person who is private-pay must be at risk of nursing home placement. These guidelines are not as intense as those during waiver since the program must build a high enough census to gain experience in managed, coordinated care. The process for participants entering into the program during this time is:

Table 15.2 Phase I: Participant Profile, July 1990 (N=37)

	Percent
Assistance with eating	60
Assistance with toileting	
0 assist	18
1 assist	68
2 assist	14
Assistance with bathing	24
Assistance with transferring	
0 assist	40
1 assist	46
2 assist	14
Wheelchairs	51
Administer medications	46
Nursing treatments	19
Dementia diagnosis	70
Wanders	14
Incontinent bowel and/or bladder	49

1. Entry point referral from the county case management agency, hospital discharge planners, or a community referral directly to the program.
2. Development and approval of eligibility both financially and functionally (utilizing the assessment tool designated by the Department of Social Services for use in determining ICF and SNF level of care for nursing home placement).
3. Assessment by the social worker or registered nurse of Total Longterm Care to determine the program's capability in meeting the needs of the participant and family members.

It is believed that the participants of TLC will be those who are the most frail since the program will accept incontinent, confused, and multiple-diagnosis participants. Other adult day care programs do not accept such individuals and typically refer them to nursing homes or back to the case management agency, a process that increases the cost to the Medicaid program. Phase I will not only add a service for the frail elderly, but it is believed by the program that there will be a decrease in overall Medicaid costs as services will be coordinated by one team instead of multiple individuals. The population currently enrolled in the program reflects the need for a program to serve the confused, incontinent, skilled individual who needs assistance with mobility, transferring, eating, and self-care within an adult day health center in the Denver area.

PHASE II: WAIVER IMPLEMENTATION

After successfully completing approximately 18 months of experience (July 1991 through December 1994) during Phase I under fee-for-service, Total Longterm Care will have negotiated a monthly capitated rate with the Health Care Financing Administration for Medicare reimbursement and with the Colorado Department of Social Services for Medicaid reimbursement. The project will have in place all appropriate mechanisms for serving the total health needs of all participants, including inpatient hospitalization, out-patient services, and nursing home contracts.

The goals of Total Longterm Care during Phase II are:

1. to successfully operate the risk-based long-term care model providing all services to the frail elderly;
2. open second and third sites within the Denver metro area;
3. increase census to adequate levels to open the third site;
4. gather statistical data to demonstrate that permanent waivers are appropriate. This data must be gathered for Medicare (specifically, the Health Care Financing Administration) and Medicaid (Colorado Department of Social Services).

This phase begins as soon as a targeted census reaches approximately 95 to 100 enrollees in the waivered program, an enrollment figure that is anticipated to be met after July 1991. By such time, the program will be certified as a home health agency in order to begin to serve participants within their homes.

Program Referral. Marketing regarding the program and services shall include community agencies; health care providers, including hospital discharge planners, nursing homes, and home health care agencies; retirement housing directors; and social groups. It is believed that a large number of referrals will be generated from the health care providers, but most especially from the point of entry at the Denver Department of Social Services and Case Management agency.

PHASE II: ARRAY OF
SERVICES, WAIVERED MODEL

The program utilizes a consolidated service model as opposed to a brokered model of case management currently used in the Colorado Home and Community-Based Services Program. The consolidated model offers the full range of medical, social, restorative, and support services to maximize the functional capacity of each participant, diminishing the need for acute care or nursing home placement. The multidisciplinary team's management of participants' needs is the core of the service model (see Figure 15.1). All caregivers (from physicians to program aides) are members of the multidisciplinary team and take part in service planning and decision-making about the care of participants.

The total health care needs of the participants will be served. There are additional services not currently reimbursed by either Medicare or Medicaid, such as dentures or home modification, that can be accessed by the multidisciplinary team in order to maintain an individual within the community. This is a strength of the modeled program. The team assesses the needs of the participants, creates the plan of care, and documents the components in the medical record. It then is responsible for providing the appropriate care directly or through contracts with other agencies. The team will then evaluate the appropriateness of the plan every 3 months to determine its effectiveness. Should a need arise between quarterly reviews, an intervention can take place within a 24-hour period since the team is able to immediately change a plan of care.

By coordinating this extensive array of medical and non-medical services, the needs of the participants are met in an out-patient environment in an adult day health center, or within their own homes or an institutional setting. This service delivery system enhances the quality of life for the participant, and serves to reduce and cap the costs for the participant's medical needs.

PHASE II: FINANCING,
WAIVERED MODEL

Risk-Based Model. The risk-based model was developed to address the needs of long-term care patients, providers, and payers. For participants, the comprehensive service package enables them to live at home

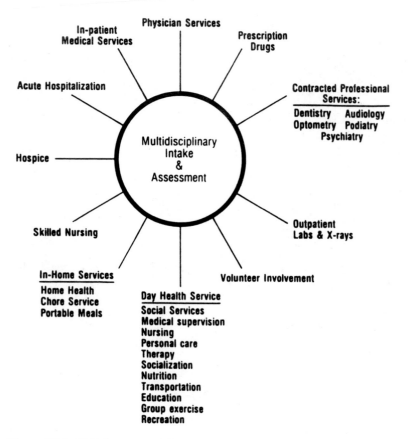

Figure 15.1. TLC Spectrum of Care Services.
SOURCE: Linda Barley, program director, TLC. Used with permission.

rather than in nursing homes. Flexible reimbursement allows providers to deliver the service participants need, rather than those services that are reimbursed in the traditional fee-for-service system. For the payers, a system is created that is less expensive since the costs are capitated. A key component to the TLC program is assuring payers (Medicare, Medicaid, and private reimbursement sources) that individuals enrolled in TLC are truly comparable to nursing home residents. Thus the assessment tool is determined by the Colorado Department of Social Services.

Monthly Capitation. At waiver implementation, the program will receive from Medicare and Medicaid a capitated monthly amount for each participant. TLC will not access the Home- and Community-Based Services program but will be a completely separate parallel waiver. Under the risk-based financing model, TLC shall assume responsibility for all costs generated by the program participants, and must begin to build a risk reserve fund that will cover any cost overages for the program. TLC is responsible for the entire range of services in this consolidated service model. At the conclusion of the demonstration period (approximately 3 years in duration), the program will assume 100% of the financial risk for the health care costs of the program participants. During Phase II, the financial risk will be shared by Total Longterm Care, Medicare, and Medicaid through a risk-sharing agreement between these agencies.

Phase II Admission Criteria. The criteria for admission to Total Longterm Care during a waiver implementation is a point of negotiation with the Colorado Department of Social Services during 1990. It is believed that all individuals over the age of 65 (required by HB 1030 and the Colorado Department of Social Services) who are functionally equivalent to the Colorado state institutionalized long-term care populations will be eligible for the program under waiver. During Phase I and prior to implementation, TLC and the Colorado Department of Social Services will enter into a contract that specifies these critical areas, along with the rate-setting methodology and risk-sharing agreement. The process for enrollment into the program is anticipated to be:

1. An entry point referral from the case management agency within the Denver metro area, hospital discharge planners, home health agencies, or from community referrals directly to the program is required.
2. A home assessment by the social worker will be conducted to determine eligibility for the program and to discuss the needs of the participant, including his or her eligibility for Medicare and Medicaid coverage.
3. If accepted into the program, the participant must elect to receive all health care services from Total Longterm Care. This includes physician services, as well as contracted services. The program cannot disenroll a participant for financial reasons but the participant may disenroll at any time.

Should a participant disenroll, he or she will return to the same services as provided by the Medicare and Medicaid programs.

Level of Care Reassessment. Once a Total Longterm Care participant meets the functional criteria as required by the long-term institutionalized population and enters the program, functional status is not reassessed for purposes of maintaining enrollment. This is different from current Home- and Communed-Based Services policy, but it is extremely important to the philosophy of the model. The health of some participants will improve enough to require a lower level of care. It is important, however, to note that these instances will be few and that many of the participants demonstrating improvement would quickly deteriorate back to eligible status if they were disenrolled. Additionally, if individuals whose conditions improve are discharged from the program, there is little incentive to increase participants' functional capacity.

PHASE III: PERMANENT WAIVERS

During calendar year 1995, Total Longterm Care must request permanent waivers for the program from the Health Care Financing Administration, the Colorado General Assembly, and the Colorado Department of Social Services. Exact parameters of this phase will be determined during the previous 5 years of experience.

Demonstration Dilemmas. As Total Longterm Care is a demonstration project, its success is yet to be measured. However, the purpose of the demonstration is to determine whether the model (On Lok replication) can succeed outside San Francisco. Populations, state environments, city geography, and cultural and generational attitudes will influence the success of the site. The proof will unfold as the Denver site continues to implement the model in its own unique way.

REFERENCES AND RESOURCES

Campion, et al. (1983). Why acute care hospitals must undertake long-term care. *New England Medical Journal,* 308.

Demographic Section, Colorado Division of Local Government. (1988, August). *Colorado Population Projections.*

Diamond, L. M., Guremberg, L. E., Morris, R. L. (1983). Eldercare for the 1980s: Health and social services in one prepaid health maintenance system. *The Gerontologist, 23* 12, 148-154.

Marine, S. (1987, September). *No simple solutions: Service delivery to the elderly in metropolitan Denver.* Denver: The Colorado Trust.

Schrier, R. W., & Lowenstein, S. W. (1982). Social and political aspects of aging. *Clinical Internal Medicine in the Aged.*

For further information, contact:

Executive Director
Total Longterm Care (TLC)
1801 E 19th Avenue
Denver, CO 80218
(303) 839-7515

References

Abrahams, R., Capitman, J. A., Leutz, W. N., & Macho, P. (1988). Case management in the S/HMO. *Generations, 12* (5), 39-43.

American Association of Retired Persons. (1988). *National survey of caregivers.* Washington, DC: Author.

American Bar Association Commission on Legal Problems of the Elderly and Commission on the Mentally Disabled. (1984). A model act regulating board and care homes: Guidelines for states. Washington, DC: U.S. Department of Health and Human Services.

Ansak, M. L. (1983). On Lok senior health services—A community care organization for dependent adults. *Pride Institute Journal of Long Term Home Health Care, 2* (1), 7-12.

Aronson, M. K., Levin, G., & Lipkowitz, R. (1984). A community-based family/patient group program for Alzheimer's disease. *The Gerontologist, 28* (5), 610-619.

Austin, C. D., & O'Connor, K. (1989). Case management: Components and program contexts. In M. D. Peterson & D. L. White (Eds.), *Health care of the elderly: An information sourcebook.* Newbury Park, CA: Sage.

Barker, J. C., Mitteness, L. S., & Wood, S. J. (1988). Gatekeeping: Residential managers and elderly tenants. *The Gerontologist, 28* (5), 610-619.

Beresford, L. (1989, October 26). San Francisco's On Lok spawns similar programs across U.S. In *LTC Management,* 4-6.

Beyer, J., Bulkley, J., & Hopkins, P. (1984). *A model act regulating board and care homes: Guidelines to states.* Washington, DC: American Bar Association, Commission on Legal Problems of the Elderly and Commission on the Mentally Disabled.

Brummel, S. W. (1984). Senior companions: An unrecognized resource for long-term care. *Pride Institute Journal of Long-Term Health Care, 3* (1), 3-13.

Capitman, J. A. (1989a). Policy and program options in community oriented long-term care. Waltham, MA: The Bigel Institute for Health Policy, Heller School, Brandeis University.

Capitman, J. A. (1989b). Present and future roles of SSI and Medicaid in funding board and care programs. In M. Moon, G. Gaberlavage & S. J. Newman (Eds.), *Preserving independence, supporting needs: The role of board and care homes.* Washington, DC: Public Policy Institute, American Association of Retired Persons.

Cohen, M. A. (1988). Life care: New options for financing and delivering long-term care. *Health Care Financing Review,* Annual Supplement, 139-143.

Cohen, M. A., Tell, E. J., Batten, H. L., & Larson, M. J. (1988). Attitudes toward joining continuing care retirement communities. *The Gerontologist, 28* (5), 637-643.

Dobkin, L. (1989). *The board and care system: A regulatory jungle.* Washington, DC: American Association of Retired Persons.

Eustis, N. N., Greenberg, J., & Patton, S. (1984). *Long-term care for older persons: A policy perspective.* Monterey, CA: Brooks/Cole Publishing.

Feder, J., & Scanlon, W. J. (1988, April). *Federal financing and fiscal incentives: Shuffling federal programs to pay for long-term care* (Pub. No. 1466-15). Washington, DC: The Urban Institute.

Feder, J., Scanlon, W. J., & Hoffman, J. (1988, August). *Board and care: Problem or solution?* Washington, DC: Center for Health Policy Studies, Georgetown University.

Firnman, J. P. (1988). Long-term care insurance: Consumer issues for an emerging industry. *Pride Institute Journal of Long Term Home Health Care, 7* (3), 3-8.

Fisher, R. S., & Donohoe, E. (1989). State regulation of adult day health care facilities. *Focus: Intergovernmental Health Policy Project, 26* (5), 1-14.

Foley, W. J. (1989, June). Holistic views of home care delivery system quality. Paper presented at National Conference on Home Care, Washington, DC.

Gaffney, J. B. (1990). National news roundup. *The Beacon, 7* (7), l.

Gwyther, L. P. (1988). Assessment: Content, purpose, outcomes. *Generations, 12* (5), 11-15.

Harrington, C., & Grant, L. (1988). *The delivery, regulation, and politics of home care: A California case study.* San Francisco: Institute of Health and Aging, University of California, December.

Hedrick, S. C., & Inui, T. S. (1986). The effectiveness and cost of home care: An information synthesis. *Health Services Research, 20* (6), Part II, 851-880.

Hereford, R. W. (1989). Developing nontraditional home-based services for the elderly. *Quality Review Bulletin, 15* (3), 92-97.

Holahan, J., & Sulvetta, M. B. (1989). Assessing Medicare reimbursement options for skilled nursing facility care. *Health Care Financing Review, 10* (3), 13-27.

Hughes, S. L. (1989). A new challenge: Assuring the quality of social services. *Generations, 13* (1), 26-30.

Institute of Medicine, Committee on Nursing Home Regulation. (1986). *Improving the quality of care in nursing homes.* Washington, DC: National Academy Press.

Johnson, S. (1988). Assuring quality of home health care for the elderly: Identifying and developing tools for enforcement. St. Louis: Center for Health Law Studies, School of Law, St. Louis University.

Joint Commission on Accreditation of Healthcare Organizations. (1988). *Standards for the accreditation of home care.* Chicago: Author.

Justice, D., Ethredge, L., Luehrs, J., & Burwell, B. (1989, April). *State long-term care reform: Development of community care systems in six states.* Health Policy Studies, National Governor's Association, Center for Policy Research, Washington, DC.

Kane, R. A., Illston, L. H., Kane, R. L., & Nyman, J. A. (1989). *Adult foster care in Oregon: Evaluation.* Minneapolis: Health Services Research and Policy School of Public Health, University of Minnesota.

Kane, R. A., & Kane, R.L. (1987). *Long-term care: Principles, programs and policies.* New York: Springer.

Kron, K., Iverson, L. H., & Pastor, B. (1989, August). The need to reform the long-term care system. *Caring,* 42-51.

Leader, S. (1987). *High tech home care.* Washington, DC: AARP Public Policy Institute.

Leutz, W. N. (1986). Long-term care for the elderly: Public dreams and private realities. *Inquiry, 223* (2), 134-140.

Leutz, W. N., Abrahams, R., Greenlick, M., Kane, R, & Prottas, J. (1988). Targeting expanded care to the aged: Early S/HMO experiences. *The Gerontologist, 28* (1), 4-17.

Lipson, D. (1988). *State financing of long-term care services for the elderly. Vol. 1 Executive Report and Vol. II State Profiles.* Washington, DC: Intergovernmental Health Policy Project, George Washington University.

Lombardi, T., Jr. (1978). *Medical malpractice insurance: A legislator's view.* Syracuse, NY: Syracuse University Press.

Luft, H. S., & Miller, R. H. (1988). Patient selection in a competitive health system. *Health Affairs, 7* (1), 97-119.

Lyons, D. (1989a, August). Long-term care case management. *Caring,* 40-41.

Lyons, D. (1989b). Long-term care case management: New opportunities result from changing trends in the finance and delivery of LTC services. Waltham, MA: LifePlans.

LTC Management. (1989a, October 26). Insurance developments, 4-6.

LTC Management. (1989b, October 31). LTC services not keeping pace with demands, 4.

Mature Market Report. (1988, October). Insurance: Life insurance enter LTC market, 4.

McCoy, J., and Conley, R. (1989). Personal communication. Washington, DC: Social Security Administration.

Miller, J. A., Berg, R. G., Bischoff, K. J., & Schlenker, R. E. (1989, September). State survey of community-based care systems: Summary of quality assurance mechanisms in sixteen states, state report from research synthesis and recommendations on the quality of selected long-term care services and on the relationship between long-term care services and reduced acute care expenditures. Denver: Center for Health Services Research, University of Colorado Health Sciences Center.

Montgomery, R. L. (1989). Respite services for family caregivers. In M. D. Peterson & D. L. White (Eds.), *Health care of the elderly: An information sourcebook.* Newbury Park, CA: Sage.

Morishita, L., Siu, A. L., Wang, R. T., Oken, C., Cadogan, M. P., & Schwartzman, L. (1989). Comprehensive geriatric care in a day hospital: A demonstration of the British model in the U.S. *The Gerontologist, 29* (3), 336-340.

Muller, C. (1989). Shared housing for the elderly. In M. D. Peterson & D. L. White (Eds.), *Health care of the elderly: An information sourcebook.* Newbury Park, CA: Sage.

National HomeCaring Council. (1988). Homemaker-home health aide services. Washington, DC: The Accreditation Program, a Division of the Foundation of Hospice and Homecare.

National League for Nursing. (1987). *Accreditation criteria, standards, and substantiating evidences.* New York: Author.

Noelker, L. S., & Bass, D. M. (1989). Home are for elderly persons: Linkage between formal and informal caregivers. *Journal of Gerontology, 44* (2), S63-S70.

Phillips, B. R., & Miller, C. (1987). *Approach to measurement of severity of illness and functioning.* Bethesda, MD: System Sciences, Inc.

Phillips, E. K., Scattergood, D. M., Fisher, M. E., & Baglioni, A. D. (1988). Public home health: Settling in after DRGs? *Nursing Economics, 6,* (1), 31-35.

Phillips, P. D., Applebaum, R. A., & Atchley, S. J. (1989). Assuring the quality of home-delivered long-term care: The Ohio quality assurance project. *Home Health Care Services Quarterly, 10* (3/4), 45-65.

Phillips, P. D., Applebaum, R. A., Atchley, S. J., & McGinnis, R. (1989). Quality assurance strategies for home-delivered long-term care. *Quality Review Bulletin, 15* (5), 156-162.

Rabin, D., & Stockton, P. (1987). *Long-term care for the elderly: A factbook.* New York: Oxford University Press.

Rechkovsky, J. D. (1989). Present and future roles of HUD programs in board and care financing. In M. Moon, G. Gaberlavage, & S. J. Newman (Eds.), *Preserving independence, supporting needs: The role of board and care homes.* Washington, DC: Public Policy Institute, American Association of Retired Persons.

Reifler, B. V., & Hansen, L. (1986). In-home mental health programs. *Generations, 10* (3), 52-53.

Riley, P. A. (1989, December). Quality assurance in home care. Washington, DC: National Academy for State Health Policy. The Center for Health Policy Development.

Rivlin, A. M., & Wiener, J. M. (1988). *Caring for the disabled elderly: Who will pay?* Washington, DC: The Brookings Institute.

Rossiter, L. F., & Langwell, K. (1988). Medicare's two systems for paying providers. *Health Affairs, 7* (2), 120-132.

Schlenker, R. F., Miller, J. A., Berg, R. G., Bischoff, K. J., & Butler, P. A. (1989, September). Future research on the quality of long-term services in community-based and custodial settings. Denver: Center for Health Services Research, University of Colorado Health Sciences Center.

Shearer, G. (1989, January). *Long-term care: Analysis of public policy options.* Washington, DC: Consumers Union.

Stanhope, M. K. (1989). Home care: Past perspectives and implications for the present and future. In C. G. Meisenheimer (Ed.), *Quality Assurance for Home Health Care.* Rockville, MD: Aspen Publishers.

Sullivan, L. W. (1989). Special report: Shattuck lecture—The health care priorities of the Bush administration. *The New England Journal of Medicine, 321* (2), 125-126.

Sykes, J. T. (1988). Living independently with neighbors who care: Strategies for enabling older residents to age in place. University of Wisconsin, Madison: Office for the Vice Chancellor, Center for Health Science.

Tell, E. J., Cohen, M. A., & Wallack, S. S. (1987). Life care at home: A new model for financing and delivering long-term care. *Inquiry, 24,* 245-252.

Upshur, C. C. (1982). An evaluation of home-based respite care. *Mental Retardation, 20* (1), 58-62.

U.S. General Accounting Office (USGAO). (1989). *Board and care: Insufficient assurance that residents' needs are identified and met.* Report to Congressional Requestors (Publication No. GAO/HRD89-50). Washington, DC: Government Printing Office.

U.S. House of Representatives. Committee on Ways and Means. (1986). *Background material and data within the jurisdiction of the Committee on Ways and Means.* Washington, DC: Government Printing Office.

U.S. Senate Special Committee on Aging. (1986). *Aging America: Trends and projections.* Washington, DC: Government Printing Office.

U.S. Senate Special Committee on Aging. (1989). *Developments in aging 1988, Volume 1.* Washington, DC: Government Printing Office.

U.S. Senate Special Committee on Aging. (1988a). *Home care at the crossroads* (Special Print 100-102). Washington, DC: Government Printing Office.

U.S. Senate Special Committee on Aging. (1988b). *The long-term care challenge: Developments in aging, Volume 3.* Washington, DC: Government Printing Office.

Vierck, E. (1990). *Paying for health care after age 65*. Santa Barbara, CA: ABC-CLIO.

Wald, F. S., Foster, Z., & Wald, H. J. (1980). The hospice movement as a health care reform. *Nursing Outlook, 28* (3), 173-178.

Weissert, W. G., & Cready, C. M. (1989). A prospective budgeting model for home- and community-based long-term care. *Inquiry, 26* (1), 116-129.

Weissert, W. G., Cready, C. M., & Pawelah, J. E. (1989). Models of adult day care: Findings from a national study. *The Gerontologist, 29* (50), 640-649.

Weissert, W. G., Cready, C. M., & Pawelah, J. E. (1990). *Adult day care: Findings from a national survey*. New York: Johns Hopkins Press.

Williams, S. J., & Torrens, P. R. (1988). *Introduction to health services*. New York: John Wiley.

Wood, J. B., & Estes, C. L. (1988). Medicalization of community services for the elderly. *Health and Social Work, 13* (1), 35-42.

Resource Associations for Community-Based Long-Term Health Care

ACTION
806 Connecticut Avenue NW
Washington, DC 20525
(202) 634-9380

Administration on Aging (AOA)
330 Independence Avenue
Cohen Building
Washington, DC 20201
(202) 245-0641

Alzheimer's Disease & Related Disorders Association
70 East Lake Street, Suite 600
Chicago, IL 60611
(312) 853-3060

American Association of Homes for the Aging (AAHA)
Suite 400, 1129 20th Street NW
Washington, DC 20036-3489
(202) 296-5960

American Association of Retired Persons (AARP)
1909 K Street
Washington, DC 20049
(202) 872-4700

American Bar Association
Commission on Legal Problems of the Elderly
Second Floor, South Lobby
1800 M. Street NW
Washington, DC 20036
(202) 331-2297

American Nurses Association
1101 14th Street NW
Washington, DC 20005
(202) 789-1800

American Society for Geriatric Dentistry
Suite 1616
211 East Chicago Avenue
Chicago, IL 60611
(312) 440-2660

American Speech, Language and Hearing Association
10801 Rockville Pike
Rockville, Maryland 20852
(301) 857-5700

Center for Health Services Research
University of Colorado Health Sciences Center
Denver, CO
(303) 756-8350

Department of Human Services
1331 H. Street NW, Suite 500
Washington, DC 20005
(202) 727-0735

Family Caring Network
LifePlans, Inc.
Two University Park
51 Sawyer Road
Waltham, MA 02154
(617) 647-3552

Foundation for Hospice and Home Care
519 C Street NE
Washington, DC 20002
(202) 547-7424

The Gerontological Society of America
1275 K Street NW, Suite 50
Washington DC 20005-4006
(202) 842-1275

Health Care Financing Administration (HCFA)
6325 Security Boulevard
Baltimore, MD 21207
(301) 594-9086

Hill-Burton Program
Health Resources and Services Administration
5600 Fishers Lane
Rockville, MD 20857
(303) 443-5656

Hospice & Home Care Accreditation Program
Joint Commission
875 North Michigan Avenue
Chicago, IL 60611
(312) 642-6061

W. K. Kellogg Foundation
400 North Avenue
Battle Creek, MI 49017-3398
(616) 986-1611

National Association of Area Agencies on Aging
Suite 208
600 Maryland Avenue SW
Washington, DC 20024
(202) 484-7520

National Association for Home Care
519 C Street NE
Washington, DC 20002
(202) 547-7424

National Association of Meal Programs
204 E Street NE
Washington, DC 20002
(202) 547-6157

National Association of RSVP Directors
2 Civic Center Plaza
El Paso, TX 79901
(202) 728-4483

National Association of State Units on Aging
Suite 304
2033 K Street NW
Washington, DC 20006
(202) 785-0707

National Association of Residential Care Facilities
1205 W. Main St., Rm. 209
Richmond, VA 23220
(804) 355-3265

National Association of Social Workers
7981 Eastern Avenue
Silver Spring, Maryland 20910
(301) 565-0333

National Committee for Quality Health Care
1730 Rhode Island Avenue, NW, Suite 803
Washington, DC 20036
(202) 861-0882

National Council on Aging
West Wing 100
600 Maryland Avenue SW
Washington, DC 20024
(202) 479-1200

National Hospice Organization
Suite 307
1901 North Fort Myer Drive
Arlington, VA 22209
(703) 243-5900

National Governor's Association
444 N. Capital St., Suite 250
Washington, DC 20001

National Institute of Adult Day Care
c/o National Council on Aging
600 Maryland Avenue SW
West Wing 100
Washington, DC 20024
(202) 749-1200

National Institute on Aging
7550 Wisconsin Avenue
Bethesda, MD 20892
(301) 496-3136

National Institute on Community-Based Long-Term Care
600 Maryland Avenue SW
West Wing 100
Washington, DC 20024
(202) 479-1200

National League for Nursing
Community Health Accreditation Program
10 Columbus Circle
New York, NY 10019-1350
(212) 582-1022

National Organization for Victim Assistance
717 D. Street NW
Washington, DC 20004
(202) 393-6682

The Robert Wood Johnson Foundation
College Road & U.S. Route 1
P.O. Box 2316
Princeton, NJ 08543-2316
(609) 452-8701

SELECT Home Health Services of America
P.O. Box 5120
Avon, CO 81620
(303) 845-0909

Senate Special Committee on Aging
Room 628 Hart Building
Washington, DC 20520
(202) 224-1467

Social Security Administration
Office of Public Inquiries
6401 Security Boulevard
Baltimore, MD 21235
(301) 594-1234

United Way of America
701 North Fairfax Street
Alexandria, VA 22314-2045
(703) 836-7100

Veterans Administration
Office of Public Affairs
810 Vermont Avenue NW
Washington, DC 20420
(202) 233-2843

Volunteers of America
3813 North Causeway Boulevard
Metairie, LA 70002
(504) 837-2652

Index

243

About the Author
and Contributors

Judith Ann Miller (Ph.D.) is self-employed in her research/writing company, Arcanum Productions, in Aurora, Colorado. She received her B.S. in education and M.S. in child development and family studies from Colorado State University, and her Ph.D. in human development and family relations/community and human services from the University of Nebraska-Lincoln. Her experiences in community-based long-term health care range from the grassroots level as executive director of a private, nonprofit home health care agency to the policymaking level at meetings in the halls of the Health Care Financing Administration. She has served as a director of an Area Agency on Aging and has a number of publications in the social service field.

John W. Abbott has been on the cutting edge of the hospice movement for the past 13 years within the Connecticut Hospice, which began hospice care in the United States in 1974. Between 1977 and 1985, he was interpretive and educational officer. He retired at the end of 1985 but continued to serve the Connecticut Hospice as a consultant; currently he is its director of public relations. He edited *Hospice Resource Manual for Local Churches,* published by Pilgrim Press in 1988. An ordained minister of the United Church of Christ, he was an executive with the National Council of Churches in New York City for many years and has served several Connecticut congregations as interim minister. A native of Redlands, California, he graduated from the University of Redlands, studied at Chicago Theological Seminary, and graduated from Andover Newton Theological School.

Robert A. Applebaum (Ph.D.) is Associate Professor in the Department of Sociology and a Research Fellow at the Scripps Gerontology Center, Miami University, Oxford, Ohio. He holds degrees from Ohio University (B.A.), Ohio State University (M.S.W.), and University of Wisconsin-Madison (Ph.D.). He has been involved in the evaluation of case management programs since 1978, working on the Wisconsin Community Care Organization, Wisconsin Community Options Program, Ohio's PASSPORT program, and the National Long-Term Care Channeling Demonstration. He has most recently been involved in the design and evaluation of a quality assurance system for Ohio's PASSPORT case management project. A frequent speaker at national and state conferences on home care, he has authored numerous articles and monographs on community-based long-term care and was the guest editor of a special issue on the topic of quality assurance, published in *Generations,* the journal of the American Society on Aging. Active in the Gerontological Society of America, he recently completed a term as book review editor of the *Gerontologist.* He also served as a member of the public policy committee, and he co-chairs the Social Research Planning and Practice task force on long-term care.

Margaret A. Auker (M.P.A.) has been the Deputy Director of the State Unit on Aging of Wyoming since 1983, where she develops and monitors the biennial budget for that state agency and contracts for statewide services. She produces bimonthly radio programs on issues facing the elderly and provides general administration to the state Agency on Aging. With an M.P.A. from the University of Wyoming, she serves as a private consultant and instructor in statistics, psychology, social work and related fields, and public administration.

Linda S. Barley (M.P.A.) is Executive Director of Total Long-term Care, Inc. She holds a bachelor's degree in psychology and a master's degree in public administration from the University of Colorado, Colorado Springs. Her involvement in the health care field extends from direct service as a Colorado licensed nursing home administrator to the development of unique Medicare certifications. She has been the administrator for an exclusive Alzheimer's disease skilled and intermediate nursing facility and for one of only twelve inpatient-only hospice programs in the country. Her community activities include an appointment to the Colorado Board of Examiners for Nursing Home Administrators, and she is co-chair of the Education Committee for the local

Denver Metro Chapter of the Alzheimer's Association. She has trained nursing home staff on both the national and statewide level on Alzheimer's disease and has assisted with the development of an Alzheimer's Association training manual.

Sharon Farley (R.N., Ph.D.) is Associate Professor at Auburn University at Montgomery School of Nursing and Director of the Rural Elderly Enhancement Program, a W. K. Kellogg Foundation project to assist the elderly in Lowndes and Wilcox counties in Alabama. She received her Nursing Diploma from St. Lukes Hospital, Cleveland, Ohio, and her B.S.N. from Ohio State University, Columbus, Ohio. After working for seven years as a pediatric nurse, she received her M.S. in maternal child health from the University of Colorado, Denver, Colorado. Her Ph.D. in nursing education administration is from the University of Texas.

Ruth Friedman (R.N., M.S.N.) is Community Respite Director for the Kellogg Respite Care Project. She came to the project from the University of Illinois College of Nursing, where she taught rehabilitation nursing as a member of the Medical-Surgical Nursing Department. She has given presentations at national workshops in rehabilitation nursing and conducted community seminars for caregivers. As a doctoral student in the Human Development and Social Policy Program at Northwestern University, she is focusing on issues of disability, aging, and social policy. Her professional affiliations include the Illinois Nurses Association, Illinois Head Trauma Association, Association of Rehabilitation Nurses and Sigma Theta Tau.

Marjorie K. Jamieson (R.N., M.S.), a nurse executive, was among six women in her community who designed and implemented the Block Nurse Program for her neighbors. She was the Volunteer Director of Services and first Chairperson of the board. She was responsible for an innovations award from Harvard University and the Ford Foundation, and for grants of 1.7 million dollars from the Division of Nursing, U.S. Department of Health and Human Services, and the W. K. Kellogg Foundation. The grants are funding replication and evaluation of the program in three social demographically diverse neighborhoods. Her undergraduate degree is from St. Olaf College. She received an M.S. in nursing administration and nursing education from the University of Minnesota.

Tarky Lombardi, Jr., a New York State Senator representing half of Onondaga County, was elected to the State Senate in 1965 and is currently serving his thirteenth term. Named Chairman of the Senate Finance Committee in January 1989, he was Chairman of the Senate Health Committee from 1971 through 1988. Responsible for the enactment of several hundred significant health-related laws, his proudest legislative accomplishment is the successful enactment and implementation of New York's Nursing Home Without Walls, which has received national acclaim. In 1985, he received the Terence Cardinal Cooke Medal for distinguished service in health care. In 1986, the National Association for Home Care honored him by naming him the state legislator whose efforts have been the most significant nationwide in the advancement of home health care. He has been named legislator of the year by many statewide organizations in recognition of his leadership and many contributions in the area of health care and human services. A graduate of New York Military Academy at Cornwall, Syracuse University, and Syracuse University School of Law, he is a member of Syracuse University's Board of Trustees.

Joan H. Moss (R.N., M.S.N.) is Project Director for the Kellogg Respite Care Project. Prior to this appointment, she was Director, Division of Nursing, American Hospital Association, and has also worked at the University of Illinois College of Nursing and the Evanston Hospital School of Nursing. During her last year of employment with the School of Nursing, she served as Faculty Development Consultant regarding the professional transition process into baccalaureate education. Her professional affiliations include the American Nurses Association, the Illinois Nurses Association, and Sigma Theta Tau. She is a Ph.D. candidate at the University of Illinois College of Nursing with a special interest in future health care trends and respite care services for the elderly.

Thomas M. Patten (M.S.W) is a native of Duluth, Minnesota, where he currently resides and is employed by Miller-Dwan Medical Center. In 1981, he and his wife opened their home to the elderly in need of long-term care. This was the beginning of what has become known as the Generations Model of Assisted Living. Today, he is director of the Generations program, where he continues new program development to apply the Generations model of community care to other populations requiring "assisted living" services, and consults with agencies wishing to replicate the Generations model.

Wanda J. Ryan (R.N., M.S., C.N.A.) is Administrator/Director of Professional Services of the Five Hospital Homebound Elderly Program. She received her master's degree in health services administration from the College of St. Francis-Joliet, Illinois, and has served as Administrator for Norrell Home Health Services and Director of Nursing for Suburban Home Health Services. She has given presentations at national workshops on such home care aspects as case management, budget impacts, and delivery of nursing care. She served as coordinator and instructor of the Home Health Management Certificate Program at the University of Illinois.

Keren Brown Wilson (Ph.D.) was one of the "principals" in the development of the first assisted living projects in Oregon. She has served as a consultant to the state of Oregon on assisted living housing; founded Concepts in Community Living, a consultant firm that provides a variety of services to congregate and assisted living facilities; and continued as an owner/operator of assisted living facilities. With an undergraduate degree from the University of Washington, an M.P.A. from Seattle University, and a Ph.D. from Portland State University, she also maintains a position as Associate Professor with the Institute on Aging at Portland State. She currently serves on a Certification Program for Housing Managers faculty for the American Association of Homes for the Aging, on the Oregon Gerontological Association board, and as Treasurer of the American Society on Aging.